Clinical Supervision in the Medical Profession

Structured reflective practice

Supervision in Context series

Clinical Supervision in the Medical Profession: Structured Reflective Practice edited by David Owen and Robin Shohet

Coaching and Mentoring Supervision: Theory and Practice by Tatiana Bachkirova, Peter Jackson and David Clutterbuck

Skills of Clinical Supervision for Nurses: A Practical Guide for Supervisees, Clinical Supervisors and Managers (Second Edition) by Meg Bond and Stevie Holland

Supervision in Action: A Relational Approach to Coaching and Consulting Supervision by Erik de Haan

Supervision in the Helping Professions (Fourth Edition) by Peter Hawkins and Robin Shohet

Psychotherapy Supervision: An Integrative Rational Approach to Psychotherapy Supervision by Maria C. Gilbert and Kenneth Evans

The Social Work Supervisor: Supervision in Community, Day Care, and Residential Settings by Allan Brown and Iain Bourne

Clinical Supervision in the Medical Profession

Structured reflective practice

Edited by

Dr David Owen and Robin Shohet

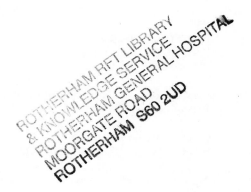

McGraw Hill

Open University Press

Open University Press
McGraw-Hill Education
McGraw-Hill House
Shoppenhangers Road
Maidenhead
Berkshire
England
SL6 2QL

email: enquiries@openup.co.uk
world wide web: www.openup.co.uk

and Two Penn Plaza, New York, NY 10121-2289, USA

First published 2012

A catalogue record of this book is available from the British Library

ISBN-10: 0-33-524292-8
ISBN-13: 978-0-33-524292-4
e-ISBN: 978-0-33-524294-8

Library of Congress Cataloging-in-Publication Data
CIP data has been applied for

Typeset by Aptara Inc., India
Printed and bound by CPI Group (UK) Ltd, Croydon, CR0 4YY

The **McGraw-Hill** Companies

Praise for this book

"I would recommend this interesting book to clinical supervisors and those involved in medical education. Doctor's roles have developed beyond patient diagnosis and treatment to helping change behaviours and involvement in the complexity of delivering healthcare, with skills in leadership, management and commissioning. The authors explore different aspects and benefits of supervision using many case based stories. However the reality is that most doctors in career grades do not benefit from any form of regular meaningful supervision and it is often only there for those undergoing training – maybe this excellent book will change that situation?"

Dr Chris Stephens, Associate Dean (Education), Faculty of Medicine, University of Southampton, UK

"This book is a significant milestone on the road to establishing reflective supervision as an essential activity for ensuring safe and ethical practice in medicine. It offers a wide range of guidance for informal and formal supervision, and for both individual and group work. The book will help to move the concept of clinical supervision for doctors from a form of instruction to a way of engaging fully with the complexities of patient care and the everyday challenges of working in the health service."

John Launer, Tavistock Clinic, London, UK

"Clinical supervision is no longer just a prop for the inexperienced or the incompetent. Neither, as the editors remind us, is it for wimps. As doctors come under ever greater scrutiny, and their work grows ever more complex, supportive yet unflinching reflection is the key if 'continuing professional development' is to be a career-nourishing experience and not just a slogan. Inspired and enthused by this book, today's professionals will welcome – even demand – opportunities to enhance their insight, skills and satisfaction through regular structured supervision."

Roger Neighbour OBE, Past President of the Royal College of General Practitioners, UK

Contents

Contributors

Christine Dunkley

Christine is a psychological therapist in secondary care in the NHS and has extensive experience of supervising mental health practitioners in multidisciplinary teams. She has written three articles on supervision for the British Association for Counselling and Psychotherapy journal. She is on the national training team for Dialectical Behaviour Therapy, a role in which she supervises psychiatrists, psychologists and nurses throughout the UK. She has been presenting workshops on supervision for seven years. She is a Senior Accredited Practitioner with BACP and an honorary lecturer for Bangor University.

Dr Helen Halpern

Helen has over twenty years' experience as a GP and for the last five years has also worked as a systemic psychotherapist, GP appraiser and medical educator. She is interested in how systemic and narrative ideas can contribute to consultations and to supervision for colleagues, trainees and patients within a rapidly changing healthcare system. Helen teaches on supervision skills courses for doctors and dentists and has helped to set up peer supervision groups to provide ongoing professional development. When not working, Helen enjoys walking with her dog, listening to music and cooking.

Dr Anita Houghton

Anita has been working in the NHS for thirty years. She is a consultant in public health and also a coach and therapist, specializing in supporting doctors and other health professionals in their careers. She is an associate of the King's Fund, and has worked closely with several other health-related organizations. She is the author of two books on career development, *Know Yourself: The Individual's Guide to Career Development in Healthcare* (Radcliffe, 2005) and *Finding Square Holes: Discover Who You Really Are and Find the Perfect Career* (Crown House Publishing, 2005) as well as numerous articles in *BMJ Career Focus* and several e-books.

Dr Sue Morrison

Sue has been working in general practice since 1979 and has been very involved in education and continuing professional development for the last twenty five years. This has included work as an NHS GP appraiser, an NHS Leadership Qualities Framework 360 facilitator, a coach–mentor and associate director with the London Deanery. Sue's particular professional interests are in coach–mentoring, supervision and interprofessional education. Her personal interests are textiles, classical singing, listening to jazz, gardening and her family.

Dr David Owen

David works in a holistic family practice and in the Faculty of Medicine at the University of Southampton where he chairs the professionalism advisory group. He provides clinical supervision to a number of GPs both individually and in groups and is a member of the Wessex Deanery tutor group training GP trainers. David trained as a supervisor with the Centre for Supervision and Team Development and has found ongoing supervision a transformative tool for his clinical work. David provides organizational and team supervision and coaching in London and the South: davidowen@doctors.net.uk.

Dr Patricia Ridsdale

Patricia is a half-time salaried general practitioner in Hampshire and also works two days a week at The Natural Practice, an integrated medicine practice in Winchester. She was a partner in a general practice for twelve years before leaving to devote more time to the complementary side of her work. She is a regular member of the Wessex Supervision Group and is a passionate advocate of the value of reflective practice for all health professionals.

Dr Paul Sackin

Paul was a GP for thirty seven years, retiring towards the end of 2010. He continues to work as a GP educator and is training programme director for the Cambridge GP training programme. He is also deputy editor of *Education for Primary Care*. Paul has been interested in Balint work ever since attending seminars run by Michael Balint himself when Paul was an undergraduate. He has led groups for many years, though currently only does so occasionally and is secretary-elect of the International Balint Federation.

Dr John Salinsky

John's favourite school subjects were English and biology. In the end biology won and John studied medicine, but always regretted the loss of literature. John continued to enjoy reading (especially the classics) and when he entered general practice, was pleased to find that characters from literature kept turning up in the surgery. A few years ago, John began writing a regular column on 'Medicine and Literature' in the journal *Education for General Practice*. John also teaches GP registrars in the Whittington Hospital vocational training scheme and has recently started to introduce the registrars to the delights of literature.

Robin Shohet

Robin has been a supervisor for thirty five years and co-founded the Centre for Supervision and Team Development (http://www.cstd.co.uk) in 1980. He is co-author with Peter Hawkins of *Supervision in the Helping Professions* (Open University Press, 4th edition, 2012), which has been translated into six languages and is used as a supervision textbook. Recent publications include *Passionate Supervision* (Jessica Kingsley Publishers, 2007) and *Supervision as Transformation* (Jessica Kingsley Publishers, 2011).

Dr Maggie Stanton

Maggie is a Consultant Clinical Psychologist heading a team of psychologists and psychological therapists in a large NHS trust. She lectures and supervises on the Doctoral Programme for Clinical Psychology and the CBT Diploma at Southampton University. She has experience of supervising professionals from a range of disciplines and runs training workshops in supervision. She is an accredited practitioner with the BABCP, a Chartered Psychologist with the British Psychological Society and a member of the Division of Clinical Psychology.

Dr Guy Undrill

Guy trained in medicine at Bristol University. After a PhD in theatre studies, he returned to medicine to become a consultant psychiatrist in Cheltenham working in acute psychiatry. His interests include motivational interviewing, risk, medical education and organizational change. He is currently a college regional adviser and the visual images editor of *The Psychiatrist*. He is a former chair of the Motivational Interviewing Network of Trainers board.

Professor Sonya Wallbank

Sonya is a Clinical Psychologist and Associate Professor of Child Health at the University of Worcester. Her clinical and research interests lie in the efficacy of clinical supervision as an intervention to aid professional well-being in the workplace. As a researcher at Leicester and Worcester Universities, she developed an interest in the quality aspects of supervision: the efficacy of the different models used as well as their utility in supporting professionals. She has delivered and evaluated supervision to a wide range of different health professionals including doctors both in the UK and the USA. She is currently working with NHS West Midlands to deliver and evaluate a regional model of clinical supervision to the health visiting workforce.

Series editor's preface

We welcome this excellent new book edited by David Owen and my colleague Robin Shohet to the Supervision in Context series. They make an excellent combination: David as medical educator and holistic family doctor, and Robin who has spent over thirty years training supervisors, including those working in medical professions. They have both contributed important chapters. While supervision has been established in many of the other helping professions such as psychotherapy, counselling, social work and psychology for several decades, the development of specific models of supervision for doctors has been much more recent. When I first consulted to hospitals thirty years ago, it was thought that a doctor having supervision indicated that they were still in training or that they had behaved unethically! Yet increasingly their demanding work requires supported reflective practice.

Doctors spend many years learning the theoretical knowledge and the technical skills necessary for medical practice. However, increasingly throughout their careers the challenging and often stressful aspects of their work come from the demanding relationships they have with their patients, colleagues – including those from different professions – managers, commissioners and regulators. Although more attention is now given to interpersonal skills in medical training than used to be the case, such training can never adequately prepare medical professionals for the wide range of relational challenges they will meet throughout their career. Supervision throughout the working life is therefore an essential part of continuing personal and professional development for all those in the medical professions.

Society is increasingly asking doctors to play a wider range of complex roles. Once the purveyors of specialist knowledge and prescriptions, doctors now have to partner their patients and coach them on their health and healthy living. This is partly because patients are much better informed by television and the internet on health matters, but also because there is a growing recognition that patients need to be active participants in their treatment. Many of the greatest causes of premature mortality result from patients' behaviour: their diet, smoking, drinking and exercise or the lack of it. Doctors are increasingly required to coach their patients on how to manage their own health better and be less reliant on chemical remedies.

Senior doctors have to manage complex businesses, whether as the clinical director of a major specialism, medical director of a Foundation Trust Hospital, acting as a director of a multi-million pound business, or managing a large general practice employing a great number of doctors, nurses, other health professionals and administrative staff.

With the introduction of Clinical Commissioning Groups, doctors are also required to manage the health economy and the difficult challenge of deciding where best to use limited resources in order to meet growing health demands and higher expectations of quality. In chapter 1 of *Supervision in the Helping Professions*, with Robin Shohet

(Open University Press, 2012), I write about the challenges of our time, particularly the limited capacity for growth while the population is increasing, especially the population over 80 who are more needy of doctors' services and while, due to the internet, everyone can access data on best quality treatment and service. The doctor as commissioner is expected to manage the gap between growing expectations and limited resources.

Today's doctors have to have great medical expertise, high standards of professional ethics and great interpersonal and relational skills with a wide variety of patients of all ages, classes and multicultural backgrounds, as well as managerial and leadership skills. Without good quality support, reflection space and continuing personal and professional development, this is an impossible challenge.

This book shows how much has changed in the last thirty years, beginning with the work of Michael Balint, who pioneered supervision and support groups for doctors. His work is written about by Paul Sackin and John Salinsky in Chapter 3. Since the work of Michael Balint, a great deal has been established in providing space for reflection and continuing personal and professional development for doctors, whether they work in primary or secondary care. This has included many forms of supervision, reflective practice and coaching. This book gives many examples of what has been, and is still being developed, as well as guidance to all medical professionals on how to ensure they get the support and development they need and guidance about how they can learn to provide it for others.

This new book sits proudly alongside the other books in this series, which include: *Supervision in the Helping Professions* by Peter Hawkins and Robin Shohet (now in its fourth edition); *Skills of Clinical Supervision for Nurses* by Meg Bond and Stevie Holland (now in its second edition); *The Social Work Supervisor* by Allan Brown and Iain Bourne; *Psychotherapy Supervision* by Maria Gilbert and Kenneth Evans; *Coaching and Mentoring Supervision: Theory and Practice* by Tatiana Bachkirova, Peter Jackson and David Clutterbuck and *Supervision in Action* by Erik de Haan. This series focuses on how to create, develop and sustain helping relationships, through providing good quality supervision to those who work broadly in the people and helping professions. Good supervision is the key link in helping practitioners connect what they learn in theory with what they learn and do in practice and is therefore the core of all continuous personal and professional development. At its best it serves and benefits the professionals who are being supervised, their clients, the organizations in which they work (and work for) and the development of the profession. In today's world no helping professional can afford to be without supervision. This book provides an excellent frame for medical students, general practitioners, hospital doctors, consultants and psychiatrists to help them know what they should demand in the way of support and supervision as part of sustaining the quality and development of their practice.

I am confident that this new publication will significantly take forward the development of supervision across the medical professions.

Professor Peter Hawkins, Series Editor

Foreword

At the beginning of the twenty-first century, people in the more affluent countries of the world find themselves living within an increasingly rules-based and bureaucratized society and subject to an ever greater degree of scrutiny and surveillance. In his book *Cosmopolis: The Hidden Agenda of Modernity,* the philosopher Stephen Toulmin dates this back to the seventeenth century:

> In choosing as the goals of Modernity an intellectual and practical agenda that set aside the tolerant, skeptical attitude of the 16th-century humanists, and focussed on the 17th-century pursuit of mathematical exactitude and logical rigor, intellectual certainty and moral purity, Europe set itself on a cultural and political road that has led both to its most striking technical successes and to its deepest human failures.
>
> (Toulmin 1990: x)

Within our contemporary healthcare system, the culmination of this great project of modernity is manifested in the ways in which individuals tend to be viewed either as units of need or as units of provision within a huge and all-embracing system. They seem always to be regarded as one or the other and the possibility that they might be both is almost never admitted. This timely book provides some much needed redress.

The great economist, philosopher and Nobel laureate Amartya Sen (2006: 26) has argued that:

> Classification is certainly cheap, but identity is not.

When people are classified on the basis of a single affiliation, be it gender, age, race or even as healthcare provider or consumer, their humanity is diminished because each of us can be described in a multitude of different ways. Sen argues that this sort of classification also has a worrying tendency to fuel conflict because difference is emphasized at the expense of what people hold in common. When doctors see patients merely as units of need, it is all too easy to regard them as demanding and unreasonable. Similarly, if doctors are there simply to provide a technical service, any degree of delay or error becomes unacceptable. All this happens much more readily in the context of the rapid erosion of continuity of care throughout the healthcare system. If doctor and patient are given the opportunity to get to know each other and to begin to trust each other, their descriptions of each other become much more detailed and conflict and misunderstanding become proportionately less likely. Clinical supervision actively encourages the clinician to consider individuals and situations from many different perspectives in order to achieve a richer understanding. This seems to echo Aristotle, quoted by Toulmin as saying:

> The Good has no universal form, regardless of the subject matter or situation: sound moral judgment always respects the detailed circumstances of specific kinds of cases.
>
> (Toulmin 1990: 31)

The American anthropologist, Clifford Geertz, famous for his espousal of 'thick description' (Geertz 1973) asks us to make the effort to see:

> particular things against the background of other particular things, deepening thus the particularity of both.
>
> (Geertz 2000: 138)

He writes:

> The contrast here is familiar, but not less important for that: between those who believe that the task of the human sciences . . . is to discover facts, set them into propositional structures, deduce laws, predict outcomes, and rationally manage social life, and those who believe that the aim of those sciences . . . is to clarify what on earth is going on among various people at various times and draw some conclusions about constraints, causes, hopes, and possibilities – the practicalities of life.
>
> (Geertz 2000: 138)

This is the task of clinical supervision, so ably laid out in this book – to help doctors and other clinicians to work out what on earth is going on between them and their patients and between them and their colleagues and to draw some conclusions about constraints, causes, hopes and possibilities – which are of course the things that make it possible to be a doctor and to be in some small way useful to patients.

Iona Heath
President, Royal College of General Practitioners

References

Geertz, C. (1973) Thick description: toward an interpretive theory of culture, in *The Interpretation of Cultures: Selected Essays*. New York: Basic Books.

Geertz, C. (2000) *Available Light: Anthropological Reflections on Philosophical Topics*. Princeton, NJ: Princeton University Press.

Toulmin, S. (1990) *Cosmopolis: The Hidden Agenda of Modernity*. Chicago, IL: University of Chicago Press.

Sen, A. (2006) *Identity and Violence: The Illusion of Destiny*. London: Penguin Books.

Preface

In the last twenty five years supervision has been increasingly seen as an important resource for the helping professions and we are delighted to be editing a book that is specifically for doctors. We view clinical supervision not as something imposed on medical professionals by their regulators, managers or those responsible for their ongoing training but rather something to be provided for and championed by doctors as something that helps them in their professional lives. In a world where pressures on many professions seem to increase almost logarithmically, it becomes harder to create the space for reflection – and yet that is when it is most needed. There is a saying that today's problems are the result of yesterday's solutions and our need for instant cures and answers could be contributing to some of the problems we face today. The quick fix is far from being quick or a fix.

As the pressures increase it becomes harder to give the time to the patient. As one doctor has described it in Chapter 1:

> I often feel that I am sitting at my desk, stuck between the lawyers behind my back with their knives out, and the computer with all the information the practice and government require me to collect in front. In this situation I feel completely alone with my fears and the expectations of others while I occasionally glimpse the patient in my peripheral vision.

Supervision helps us to bring the patient back into focus – not just their illness, but the context in which doctor and patient both meet. The quality of the supervisory relationship can both act as a mirror for the patient/doctor relationship and give opportunities to see the interactions with patients from a new perspective. Many supervisees have found this not only a way of reviewing a 'difficult case' or formalizing and developing their reflective capacity but also a transforming and liberating experience. Supervision certainly can be something you do to put things right, restore things, address problems, but it can also sharpen our clinical edge and encourage us to step more fully into the mastery of our practice and release our wisdom.

This need for reflective space, which we believe is central to maintaining a fresh approach to our work, is met by clinical supervision. Michael Carroll (2011) talks about heroes of learning who do not shirk challenges and have the ability to step back and pose hard questions about why things are done this way and how they could be done differently. Doctors are accomplished learners. They would not have got as far as they have if they were not. But the learning that supervision invites is perhaps of a different kind. It is an ability and willingness to stay open even when everything in the system, ourselves and colleagues is asking us to play safe, close down, practise defensively and protect ourselves. Supervision as we champion it asks you to hold the ability to be both vulnerable and authentic – it is not for wimps! We see it as part of the journey of lifelong learning, different from informational learning, a learning that is done through relationship and particularly the supervisory relationship.

In the first chapter we describe what we mean by clinical supervision and this is followed by a map of supervision, the five realms, that can be applied across models and disciplines. In Chapter 3 we read about the Balint group, one of the earliest forms of supervision for doctors. In Chapter 4 the authors write about a model of supervision, narrative supervision that has been widely trialled by the London Deanery. Chapters 5 and 6, incidental supervision and peer supervision, describe supervision in less formal settings. Chapter 7 looks in more depth at the benefits of supervision for the doctor's well-being. Chapter 8 is about coaching, an increasingly popular addition to forms of reflective practice. In Chapter 9 the authors describe how appraisal can be used as a form of supervision and in Chapter 10 we include a look at the evidence for supervision. Chapter 11 is written from a supervisee's perspective and finally, in Chapter 12, the topic of resistance to and in supervision is discussed.

The contributors come from a variety of backgrounds and we have ourselves learnt from the different approaches included in this book. Rather than introduce each chapter now we have asked each author to give an overview and we ourselves have written a short piece that we hope will contextualize their chapter. As experienced supervisors and trainers, our intention in gathering together similarly experienced people is to put supervision for doctors more on the map. There may come a time when its benefits will be so recognized that not to have it will be considered as old fashioned as not using technology to assist diagnosis. And as one supervisee said to us, 'I hope it becomes as important a part of everyday practice as washing your hands.'

Our underlying motive for compiling this book has been to encourage more doctors to take part in and develop their reflective capacity, and to offer and receive supervision. We have chosen to do this as an edited book as we wanted as many different voices as we could to be included. Our wish is that you benefit from their collective wisdom.

David Owen and Robin Shohet

Reference

Carroll, M. (2011) Supervision: a journey of lifelong learning, in R. Shohet (ed.) *Supervision as Transformation*. London: Jessica Kingsley Publishers.

Acknowledgements

Many people have helped and supported us in this project. The contributors in the book, without whom there would have been no book, were willing to give up time and come together to meet each other to share ideas. John Launer at the very beginning of our project came and gave us his time when we had no clear idea of the form the book would take. Joan Wilmot, and in the final stages Christine Dunkley, gave invaluable feedback and were both very generous with their time. And finally Peter Hawkins, as series editor, gave us many useful suggestions which we have incorporated.

For David it is my medical colleagues, especially Lee, with whom I first discovered I could learn more from my difficult cases than the easy ones. Also to Alice, Charles, Brian, Andy and David with whom I first sat and explored supervision with Robin. Thank you Robin as a supervisor, friend and editor who is always encouraging me to look below the surface. And other members of the Centre for Supervision and Team Development for their excellent supervision training and openness to all professional groups. To Faith Hill and Chris Stephens who have encouraged my work in medical education and enabled me to see the relevance of clinical supervision for doctors. To my father, who like many, endured an era of medical practice where their personal well-being was low on the list of anyone's priorities, but who remained open and caring to those in need regardless of the price. Finally to my son, William, who has given feedback on my writing and who I hope may practise medicine in an era where the supervision we write about is the norm.

For Robin it is my colleagues in the Centre for Supervision and Team Development, Peter Hawkins, Judy Ryde and Joan Wilmot with whom I have devised supervision courses and co-supervised for thirty five years. Thank you, David, for moving from supervisee to friend and inspiring colleague. And finally a huge appreciation to my family who push me to live the insights I gain from supervision, and especially to Joan whose intuition and discerning eye I count on.

1 Introduction to clinical supervision

David Owen and Robin Shohet

Editors' introduction

In this chapter we offer a comprehensive definition of supervision taken from Hawkins and Shohet's *Supervision in the Helping Professions* (2012) and discuss its relevance to the medical profession. We recognize that supervision can mean many things to different people. Our aim has been to clarify how the term is used and to differentiate clinical supervision from educational and managerial supervision so that its value and relevance can be recognized whatever the background, speciality or career stage of the doctor. This chapter introduces some basic principles of supervision and looks at supervision from a number of different perspectives. We show how clinical supervision builds on reflective practice and illustrate how the authors use clinical supervision in practice. It goes on to explore the potential benefits of clinical supervision throughout a doctor's career and puts in context other chapters in the book.

Overview of chapter

The medical profession is always seeking to improve patient care, look after its practitioners and increase efficiency of services. Our belief is that supervision has an important part to play in this. In this chapter, we share our perspectives on the different kinds of supervision, and focus specifically on clinical supervision and its benefits. The chapter is an orientation for the rest of the book, and it will be useful for those thinking about starting supervision, as well as those more used to giving and receiving supervision.

Introduction

In this chapter we explore how regular ongoing clinical supervision can become a cornerstone for maintaining a doctor's clinical work. We see clinical supervision as a resource that doctors can make use of throughout their professional life; a resource which can contribute to personal resilience and well-being as well as to the practical challenges that every clinician regularly faces.

We promote an eclectic approach to clinical supervision that complements the educational supervision to which many doctors already have access. We intentionally focus on clinical supervision as it relates to regular ongoing clinical practice although much of what is offered is equally relevant to clinical supervision of trainees. For many doctors 'clinical supervision' is associated with the supervisor knowing best and telling the supervisee what is right (*super*-vision, where the supervisor 'oversees' the supervisee). We describe in this book several models of clinical supervision that provide an opportunity for supervisees to 'look anew' at what challenges them, where the supervisor works to 'enable and empower' the supervisee to address clinical dilemmas. (Super-*vision*, where the supervisor helps the supervisee to see issues from a different perspective.)

Supervision describes a number of different types of encounter practitioners may have with another professional to enable their learning, development and support. Although the concept, language and style of supervision as we are using it may be foreign to some doctors, many of the activities of supervision already happen for doctors in a number of different settings such as case discussions, significant event analysis, appraisal, training, meetings with a mentor, practice meetings, or even just informal conversations (see Chapters 5 and 6). Many doctors experience supervision as a trainee and some have regular clinical supervision, for example trainee psychiatrists when they are delivering therapy. We suggest in this book ways that both doctors and patients will benefit through doctors having regular ongoing supervision.

What is clinical supervision?

The following is taken from the fourth edition of *Supervision in the Helping Professions* (Hawkins and Shohet 2012).

> Supervision is a joint endeavour in which a practitioner with the help of a supervisor, attends to their clients,[1] themselves as part of their client practitioner relationships and the wider systemic context, and by so doing improves the quality of their work, transforms their client relationships, continuously develops themselves, their practice and the wider profession.

We recognize that the above is a long and complex definition, but we consider it essential to understand how supervision is a complex task which sets out to serve a number of key stakeholders. At a minimum supervision should be in service of:

- the learning and development of the supervisee;
- the patients of the supervisee and the quality of service they receive;

- the organization(s) that employ the supervisee and the effectiveness and efficiency of the organization's work;
- the ongoing learning and development of the profession in which the supervisee and, possibly, the supervisor work.

Done well, we believe that supervision can and should serve four or more masters. To better understand this definition we will look at each phrase:

Supervision is a joint endeavour: it is important that supervision is not seen as an activity done by the supervisor on the supervisee. Both the supervisee and the supervisor need to be working in partnership, standing shoulder to shoulder facing the challenges of the work, within a clear contract in service of the supervisee and the wider system.

... **in which a practitioner with the help of a supervisor, attends to their clients:** supervision always involves patients, otherwise it becomes a form of counselling at work. It provides the opportunity for supervisees to stand back and reflect on each of their patients so as to understand the patients better and what might best help them.

... **themselves as part of their client practitioner relationships:** we believe that an objective understanding of the patient is neither achievable or desirable but practitioners need to understand the patient in the context of their professional relationship, which entails reflecting on themselves as part of the relational context.

... **and the wider systemic context:** the relationships with the patients never exist in isolation, but always in a systemic context, which includes the organizational and professional context, the wider social and political context in which the organization operates, as well as the family and social context of the patient.

... **and by so doing improves the quality of their work, transforms their client relationships, continuously develops themselves, their practice and the wider profession:** supervision is not just a reflective process but one that needs to produce learning and improvement outcomes for supervisees, their patients, their future practice, the organization and the profession.

As the above indicates, being in clinical practice means taking into account multiple points of view. Sometimes we have to try and 'see things through the patient's eyes'; at other times we need to maintain a very clearly objective perception. Moving between these perspectives is part of the 'art of medicine'. One aspect of clinical supervision is reflecting on these different perspectives, identifying which is the most appropriate in any one setting and supporting the doctor who has to hold perspectives that do not 'sit easily' with them. The case that Emma, a general practitioner, brought to supervision illustrates this.

CASE EXAMPLE: EMMA

Emma is treating a man age 59 who has metastatic prostate disease. He had discussed with Emma his impotence secondary to hormonal treatment. He mentioned that he has not had sex with his wife for some time but that he is having an affair and is considering stopping his hormonal treatment. Emma is also treating his wife, who does not know about the affair. Emma describes feeling 'weighed down' by the secret she is carrying and also a 'little angry' with the husband. In supervision she is able to review the treatment and advice she has given, which is completely appropriate. She is able to look at why she is angry and to let out that it is more than 'a little anger' she feels. She feels taken advantage of and resents the husband, and she can recognize to some extent she holds this position as a surrogate on behalf of the wife. She is concerned that she will in some way breach the husband's confidentiality and talking about it enables her to see that part of her wants the wife to find out. She is anxious that if the husband dies, the wife will find out and challenge Emma about what she knew of the husband's affair. In talking it through, issues about confidentiality, including the principle that confidentiality is maintained even following the patient's death, helped Emma clarify how she will manage her own attitude to 'the secret'. In supervision Emma was able to rehearse what she would say to the husband next time he consults her. At a subsequent meeting Emma commented that because of the supervision she had felt able to respond differently to the husband and better about seeing his wife.

Tensions arising from seeing things from many different perspectives and conflicting priorities exist not just between doctors and patients, but also between the views and priorities of colleagues, different work environments, purchasing groups, professional organizations and even the government. In many instances doctors will be clear about the course of action that the situation requires, but sometimes they will have to manage their own uncertainty about what they should do, how they should do it, how to do it with the resources available or even how they feel about doing it, given these multiple perspectives which may conflict.

Doctors with high workloads, time pressures and administrative overload have every right to claim a space for themselves, to slow down, think in more detail about a case, brainstorm solutions, express their opinions and frustrations while exploring their own creativity. In addition they can ask for feedback, identify areas in which they want to improve and connect with their vulnerability. Clinical supervision provides an opportunity to do this. It poses important questions which are helpful to consider. As one doctor commented,

> So much is about my attitudes and awareness – when these are transformed my way of working and my effectiveness are also transformed. It takes courage to show my work with honesty – the highs and the lows . . . Supervision gently illuminates my blind spots and monitors my safety and the safety of my patients.

Central to doing this is the safety of the supervisory relationship, which we explore later under contracting.

Benefits of clinical supervision

Clinical supervision offers practical ideas that can be tried and rehearsed in the supervision setting and provides a space for facilitated reflection, both of which we have found contribute to well-being. There is an opportunity to look deeply at why a particular issue has occurred, its relevance to the supervisee and the connection between an individual's experience of a particular issue and the provision of care. Over the years of supervising and training supervisors we have found that patients benefit when doctors meet their own well-being needs (see Chapter 7) and have opportunities for personal and professional development. We foresee an opportunity for regular, ongoing clinical supervision to build on the more positive aspects of appraisal and reflective practice (see Chapter 9). We have found that regular supervision can improve the quality of the clinical relationship, itself a predictor of patient care and outcome. Supervision can contribute to breaking the cycle of stress and burnout (Nielsen and Tulinius 2009) that doctors are susceptible to and that might themselves be linked to making errors (West *et al.* 2006). In addition, supervision provides a structured reflective space to review management and care decisions, ethical issues and the relationship between patient, doctor and other members of the healthcare team. All these can impact on patient care and service provision. While few doctors currently have the opportunity to avail themselves of this sort of supportive supervision, we envisage a time when doctors will not only consider it their right to have access to such support, but will see it as integral to maintaining their personal well-being and professional persona. Many readers will be familiar with the feelings, when they hear about colleagues in difficulty, of 'there but for the grace of God go I', or, 'it could easily have happened to me' and, 'it's just a matter of time'. These common refrains when hearing doctors talking about colleagues in difficulty point towards the fear doctors have of what might happen to them. When we have talked to medical professionals about what is currently available in the way of support, especially through revalidation and appraisal, we detect in many a sense of disempowerment ('more hoops to jump through'), that doctors feel vulnerable ('better keep my head down and not own up that I need support') or defeatism ('it won't stop the next Shipman'), or even a cynicism which increases as the gap widens between the reality experienced and the beliefs held ('just tell them what they want to hear'). Our experience is that when doctors are supported through clinical supervision they are able to move beyond the feelings mentioned above. They start to get their individual needs met and address more positively their continued professional development (see Chapter 12). It is not a question of either keeping up to date or getting support, but of both working synergistically.

There is a slowly growing awareness that clinical supervision can make an ongoing contribution, as part of everyday professional life, throughout a medical professional's career regardless of the doctor's speciality (see Chapter 10 for a survey of the research). This in turn could address some of the cultural and organizational challenges that a modern healthcare system wrestles with. Colleagues we have supervised often comment on their high level of stress and the impact this is having not just on them but also those around them – patients, colleagues and family. As one supervisee commented, his spouse thought he had become 'hardened' and 'withdrawn' since starting in a new job, but this was just his way of 'protecting' himself.

The doctor and patient communicate with each other on many levels and difficulties arise when aspects of the patient are not noticed or addressed by the doctor. Noticing what would otherwise go unnoticed and addressing what would otherwise be left out are part of the reflective process we are advocating in this book. For example, a doctor reflecting on a significant event may recall information from the notes or from previous meetings that he or she had not recognized at the time of the event. Equally this information may only surface after discussing the case with colleagues who had also seen the patient. Sometimes a significant event analysis will reveal aspects of our work we wish to have further training in or where we might proceed more cautiously. At other times we may remain unclear about what happened to cause a problem or uncertain how we would act differently. These are like blind spots that, until someone else helps us 'see' them clearly, are likely to remain unchanged. We each have our own individual 'blind spots' and areas we struggle to see or interpret clearly, and it is perceiving and exploring these that is so enhanced by clinical supervision. This in turn increases our ability to perceive patients more fully. Recognizing that we will all encounter situations that we are unsure about in which we will have to face our limits and uncertainty is part of professional maturity. This will help us in resolving important issues that may affect us in a way we do not initially understand or that we find difficult to manage. Such situations often include those patients we perceive as 'dumping' on us, those becoming dependent on us and so-called heartsink patients. It is often these patients that take up a lot of our time. Reframing them from individuals and situations that cause us problems to ones from which we have much to learn is often a key skill of those who seek to use clinical supervision regularly.

Roger's case below illustrates how supervision supports doctors and can address feelings in the supervisee that need a time and place to be worked through, allowing reflection about what lies behind these feelings and the wider implications for clinical practice.

CASE EXAMPLE: ROGER

Roger is in one-to-one supervision and says that he keeps thinking about a patient he saw recently and he can't 'get her out of his head'. He talks about a Rwandan woman who consulted with him a few weeks ago. Since seeing her, the doctor has on several occasions had 'flashbacks' to the brutal torture the patient described of herself and of her relatives that were 'lost'. The doctor is able to let some of his feelings out in a 'safe place' although he feels powerless and vulnerable when thinking about this event, and this is mirrored by his powerlessness to control when these thoughts 'catch him out'. Roger is invited to talk about what particular part of the patient's narrative evokes the strongest feelings in him. He talks about how the patient's father had negotiated with those who were going to kill him and his family. Tears come to the doctor's eyes when talking about the father offering to pay his attackers to shoot him and his sons rather than club them to death. The patient witnessed the atrocity but was powerless to intervene and was the only family member to survive. Roger is encouraged to explore when else he has similar feelings of powerlessness and vulnerability. He talks about his powerlessness to 'make things better' for this patient and other patients. He goes on to get in touch with his vulnerability in relation to making time from his busy job to see his own children and the 'impossible choices a father has to make'. At the same time Roger is able to see that anyone would have been traumatized by hearing of these events but that it was difficult to recognize this at the time perhaps because his role of supporting the patient conflicts with his own emotional reaction to what he is hearing. Supervision helps him get in touch with his feelings and explore ways of managing his own vulnerability and powerlessness when having to also care for a patient. At a subsequent supervision session he mentions the 'flashbacks' have stopped and he feels grateful for what he learnt from his patient.

Educational and managerial supervision

There are overlaps and similarities between educational, managerial and clinical supervision but the emphasis and orientation of the supervision, role and experience of the supervisor and expectations and selection of issues to bring by the supervisee differ considerably. Educational supervision focuses on imparting knowledge and assessment (Launer 2006), while managerial (sometimes called administrative or normative) supervision often focuses on specific targets and performance.

Educational supervision

When the purpose is predominantly educational, then supervision complements an individual's formal education. It plays a valuable role in moving theoretical understanding into practical competences. Educational supervision aims to develop 'best practice' with the help of a more experienced colleague that may be a tutor, mentor or role model. Students and junior doctors may look to more senior colleagues for guidance, and the strong and important 'formative' influence of this in forming the professional persona is well recognized (Kenny *et al.* 2003). Educational supervision may be part of developing professional artistry in conjunction with technical mastery, and provide an opportunity to explore the importance of feelings, including their central importance to learning experiences in early clinical years (Foster 2009). The educational supervisor, when able to look beyond a curriculum and respond to a supervisee's individual learning needs, plays a major role in enabling a trainee's learning and development (Kennedy 2009) to be situated within a context of professional community (Lave and Wenger 1991). In the right setting educational supervision helps participants to understand the perspective of the training establishment or regulatory body and how this shapes their relationship to their professional community.

Managerial supervision

Managerial supervision is often primarily about maintaining standards and co-ordinating practice with policies or guidelines. It is a powerful tool in exploring and developing clinical practice, using personal and professional resources efficiently and helping individuals and teams recognize and develop procedures and protocols. With an emphasis on 'quality control' and 'efficiency' it plays a part in recognizing the importance to performance of individual and team well-being and support. A key aspect of managerial supervision is to explicitly balance the emphasis between organizational goals and the supervisee's individual needs. Managerial supervision is often provided to teams and is referred to as team supervision that may be provided by a member of the team, a manager or an independent facilitator or supervisor. It can significantly help individuals and teams to address performance problems, tensions between team members (or their roles), issues with guidelines, protocols or other 'red tape' and problems when individual and organizational values are not aligned. The emphasis, as with some forms of coaching, is often on the task that needs doing. The managerial supervisor aims to 'normalize' a doctor's behaviour and actions for a particular team or organization. While a good manager may well have the clinical needs of the patient and the educational needs of the doctor in mind, their emphasis is often on monitoring the work of those they manage and improving the work towards the targets (or guidelines) of the practice or organization they are appointed by.

Clinical supervision

In clinical supervision the main external reference is the clinical relationship between patient and doctor. Although it is mainly about the work with patients it also includes the work environment. Whether the issue is between the supervisee and a particular patient or between the supervisee and a work colleague, the reference point is – 'How does this impact on the supervisee's ability to care for and treat patients?' Clinical supervision supports and holds the supervisee, provides a 'restorative' function (Proctor 2001) to assist the supervisee in managing challenges and promotes resilience. Clinical supervision tolerates uncertainty (Mollon 1989) while providing an opportunity for doctors to restore their equilibrium and rehearse how they can manage situations differently. Although the emphasis will be different depending on whether there is primarily a managerial, educative or clinical purpose to the supervision, in practice the different functions of supervision can be, and often are, combined in any supervision process. At times the relationship between the supervisor and supervisee will need to shift slightly to enable the different functions to be attended to and this is covered by the contracting process and supervisory relationship.

Individual or group supervision

A supervisee may work one-to-one with a supervisor in individual supervision, or as part of a group of individuals or part of a team. Individual and group supervision have much in common but also some important differences. In group supervision participants have to share the time available to present their work or issue but often the material one person brings is extremely informative and helpful to others. Group supervision can be cost-efficient and provide collegiate support. Group supervisors should be knowledgeable about group dynamics and how to manage groups, especially as more challenging issues can affect the way a group behaves. In experienced hands bringing the attention of a group to this change in behaviour can provide an additional resource for the supervisor and group.

Contracting and the supervisory agreement

The agreement between supervisor and supervisee sets the ground rules for the supervision process and the tone for the supervisory relationship. It provides both explicit and implicit points of agreement and processes for working through common difficulties. Unless the supervisee is very experienced it is normally the supervisor that takes the lead in initiating such aspects of the agreement. While the supervisor may initiate the discussion, it is important to realize the agreement is a dynamic one that unfolds and shifts over time to reflect the supervisee's needs.

In all supervision there are third parties that influence the work that is done. How this is dealt with is established in the contract, and includes looking at issues of boundaries, confidentiality and consent. In educational supervision the third party is usually a training or regulatory establishment. In managerial supervision it is the team or organization that the doctor works in or for. While in clinical supervision it is the clinical care of the patient that is primary, and this can extend to relationships with colleagues and the well-being and resilience of the doctor (Burton and Launer 2003). Each has its place and works with real-life encounters with patients or colleagues but in each the intention is different.

Clinical supervision relies greatly on the relationship and agreement between supervisee and supervisor. It is ultimately the quality of this relationship and the agreement between supervisor and supervisee that determines whether supervision is effective or not. Hunt suggests that there needs to be a degree of warmth, trust and genuineness and respect between them (supervisor and supervisee) in order to create a safe enough environment for supervision to take place (Hunt 1986). The quality of the supervisory relationship needs to be sufficiently open, clear and responsive to allow the supervisee to present all aspects of his or her relationship with the patient, while at the same time to be able to explore the dynamic between the supervisee and the supervisor. An important part of what the supervisor does is to enable the supervisee to be more fully aware of what actually takes place in the supervision session, as this often mirrors what happens between the doctor and patient. For example, one supervisee, Jane, came to supervision with feelings of being persecuted by patients and working defensively. Jane commented:

> I often feel that I am sitting at my desk, stuck between the lawyers behind my back with their knives out, and the computer with all the information the practice and government require me to collect in front. In this situation I feel completely alone with my fears and the expectations of others while I occasionally glimpse the patient in my peripheral vision.

A conversation about the supervisory agreement that looked at confidentiality and consent brought out Jane's fear that the supervisor was 'judging her' and that she could only 'open up so far'. Once Jane and the supervisor had agreed on confidentiality and consent Jane was invited to reflect how she felt now, recounting her feelings. She felt vulnerable and uncertain about what the supervisor would think about her – even that he might 'report her' (this is an example of parallel process described in Chapter 2). By focusing on her feelings in supervision Jane recognized that they mirrored the feelings she had in her consulting room with a few dissatisfied patients. Jane explored what she needed to do differently with these patients and thought explaining to the patient about confidentiality and consent would help. After really 'letting this sink in' and being able to talk about managing patients' dissatisfaction, and her own and her patients' (unrealistic) expectations, she was able to understand her insecurities and fears.

The difference between reflective practice and supervision

If reflective practice is considered an intelligent conversation with oneself, then clinical supervision, on the other hand, is an intelligent conversation with another about a case or issue (Launer 2003). Reflective practice provides an opportunity to run through again, in our 'mind's eye', what happened. It looks at the events 'reflected' in the mirror of our past experience and learning. Supervision in many ways starts from, nurtures and extends reflective practice. It encourages using reflective questions, not just during supervision but also as a regular part of managing challenging situations and consultations – such as, What do I think worked well? What questions are unanswered by this encounter? How do I imagine the patient or a colleague might comment on this interaction? What have I been left feeling and why? The asking of good questions is central to all types of supervision, reflective practice and coaching (see Chapters 4 and 8).

However, reflective practice on its own may leave unresolved some issues and feelings, and fail to explore fully patterns that repeat or raise questions the doctor is avoiding. Self-reflection can help us manage and cope with many challenges, puzzles and disappointments. However, if a reflective process is likened to seeing yourself in a mirror, then reflection may not, like a mirror, reveal what is under the surface of what is seen (Johns 1999), or even that the mirror itself may be distorted. Neither does reflection address assumptions or interpretations of what is being seen or avoided. To really gain insight into why certain issues reoccur for us or why certain 'buttons get pushed' often requires a separate point of reference, which a supervisor provides. Supervision brings an additional objectivity and may be thought of as holding an overviewing position. It is this perspective that distinguishes the process as 'supervision'. Ideally someone who is able to view the supervisee and her work objectively provides supervision but at the same time the supervisee needs to feel confident the supervisor can empathize with her and can appreciate the context in which she works. Supervision by an immediate peer can help to move on from a completely personal reflective process but may lack the objectivity and challenge that an external supervisor brings.

Sometimes the challenge that supervision brings is very different from how reflection works, as the supervision of Jane illustrates.

CASE EXAMPLE: JANE

Jane was taking part in a group supervision that met for five days a year. When asked if there was a case or issue she wished to bring for supervision she initially said there was not anything too important. She went on to speak about how busy she was and discussed an issue related to time management. Later as the group was about to break for lunch Jane mentioned she really could do with some help with a very difficult patient. This patient was a registered drug addict with low self-esteem and always seemed to arrive at the most awkward time (like the time the issue surfaced in the group – just before lunch) with a deeply distressing complaint that Jane felt she was unlikely to be able to help with. There was an urgency and desperateness in Jane's voice when she was talking about the patient and it evoked a desire in the group to support her. Jane described feeling tense talking about it and thought others in the group must be thinking her not good enough (like her patient). She commented she had reflected on why this patient was 'difficult' and had some strategies to cope but she seemed to have 'lots of patients like this and just couldn't go on'. The supervisor felt uncertain about addressing this case just before lunch and he pointed out that this case had not been mentioned earlier and the group was being put in a similar situation to the one Jane had been put in by the patient. The supervisor noticed his own feelings of uncertainty and being overwhelmed given how and when the issue surfaced. While acknowledging Jane's obvious distress the supervisor shared his own feelings and invited Jane to reflect on whether these feelings mirrored her own in some way. Jane said they did. Despite Jane obviously being distressed, the supervisor felt that if they started this work with such poor contracting over time, then clarity and insight would be unlikely. Instead, he recommended they 'park the issue' and the group broke for lunch. That afternoon Jane was quiet and did not bring the case up again. Jane missed the next two groups and two members expressed disappointment that the group had not helped her (in a way the group was continuing to support Jane even in her absence). When she next came she shared that she had got significant insights from the group into how she was being sabotaged by patients like the one she presented (and that had been enacted in her dynamic with the group and supervisor). She went on to talk about why she worked so much with drug addicts and insights she had had on how to balance this work better with her other commitments. She commented that the supervisor and group making a choice not to deal with an issue 'just before lunch' modelled for her the ability to make some choices. Jane commented on being more aware of the 'distressing content' of her work and the need for a time and place for relaxation. Interestingly, her relationship with the patient had changed as he picked up her improved clarity around boundaries.

This is an example of how the supervisor was able to model a way of being around boundaries that carried over into the supervisee's practice.

Ongoing clinical supervision

Ongoing supervision throughout one's professional career has developed as an integral part of most of the caring and helping professions. In these professions it is a cornerstone of professional practice with regular protected time and resources. While many doctors recognize the value of supervision in training or as part of a remedial process, few see it playing a key role in their ongoing day-to-day professional practice (see Chapter 9). There are, of course, many external reasons why it is difficult for doctors to access regular ongoing clinical supervision once they have completed their training, such as lack of time, potential cost and lack of clinical supervisors. Talking to those who do use regular supervision, there is a sense that at some level that is not unique to doctors, it is difficult to engage with those things we find most challenging. For doctors perhaps it sits uneasily with the 'hero' or 'warrior' role that doctors have to develop – the 'hero' that daily supports patients who are distressed and facing major life events and the 'warrior' who battles against debilitating disease, having to make tough choices about life and death decisions. Perhaps in this environment it is difficult for doctors to sit with feelings of uncertainty, and even hard for patients to realize that doctors need help and support at times. It is understandable that those who wish to avoid this discomfort might find different reasons to avoid a process that brings these feelings to their attention. They may prefer instead to keep focused on the task in hand, creating a work pattern where there is no time for this reflective process, or trying to steer their work away from areas that remind them of their uncertainty (for a fuller discusssion see the final chapter). In many situations doctors have developed strategies (some might say survival strategies in the complaints, fitness to practise and litigious environment in which we practise) to protect themselves from the diverse views, expectations and projections of others, whether colleagues, patients, managers or regulators.

Ongoing supervision offers an opportunity to examine when and how the different defences we set up (each at a cost to us and our work) are useful. While some are healthy coping mechanisms to the many challenges of medical practice, others when inappropriately held may jeopardize the care patients receive, threaten the well-being of doctors, or hold back professional development (see Chapter 9). For example, one aspect of the doctor–patient relationship that commonly surfaces in supervision of doctors is around issues to do with unrealistic expectations of the patient. This sometimes reflects patients' expectation of the doctor: 'But you always know what is best' or 'Just make me better' (with, of course, its shadow – to be held responsible for what goes wrong). At other times it reflects doctors' feelings that they must always have the answer (or the shadow – 'whatever I do is not going to be enough'). This potent mix of idealization and unrealistic expectation makes it hard for doctors to ask for, and receive, regular support as they may have bought into the idea that they should know best. Once seen for what they are, the pressures from idealization and unrealistic expectations, to name just two ingrained beliefs, can be managed with more insight.

As you might expect, the sorts of issues and insights one brings to or gets through supervision depend in part on the frequency and context in which supervision takes place. The insights available when the focus is as a one-off session looking at a specific problem are quite different from those that emerge in a course of supervision that invites reflection on all aspects of practice, which are again different from what emerges in supervision as part of an ongoing career-long process. For many, the first awareness that there is a process available to them for support and development is in itself a significant breakthrough, as the example of Ruth illustrates.

CASE EXAMPLE: RUTH

Ruth attended a course of four half days on supervision for doctors. In the initial session she wanted to concentrate on the different interventions that doctors in the group used when a 'difficult to manage' hypertensive patient presented. 'What would you do?' she challenged others in the group. After presenting a case at the second session where whatever advice was offered by the group was 'not good enough', the supervisor invited Ruth to talk about what it felt like when nothing was good enough. (An individual will often project onto others what they are feeling.) Ruth was able to notice that she often had the feeling of 'not being good enough' for the patient. She went on to say that she had the same feeling that she was not as good as others in the group and that she was thinking of leaving. Exploring this more, Ruth talked about feeling that whatever she did it was never enough. The supervisor invited the group members to comment on what they were feeling at this point. Several members resonated with what Ruth felt and many felt alone with the pressure of patients and their own expectations. (Usually an issue will touch several, if not all members of a group even though one person initially brings it.) One member commented that she often finds it 'easier just to get on with things on my own than ask for help'. The group including Ruth went on to explore their fear of failure and how this fear was initially intensified rather than relieved when they asked for help. It was as if the fear of asking for help had covered up or displaced the fear of failure. Interestingly the next case Ruth brought to supervision was one where she felt she had done something wrong rather than one where she might 'just have done better'. Invited to reflect on this she commented that she felt it was now all right to ask for help as others had also shown their vulnerability and she realized she had always felt her training was about 'being strong'.

While many doctors are exquisitely compassionate, sensitive and alert to their patients' needs, our experience is that they rarely focus these attributes on themselves or even colleagues. Under a banner of continued professional development a number of attributes and values have been championed to improve the safety and care of patients, but time is seldom made to bring the same humanistic and person-centred values and attributes to bear on their own and colleagues' lives, or to examine the impact of their work on their relationship to family and loved ones. Ongoing supervision allows such issues to be addressed.

Often it is only as we develop our clinical experience beyond our basic training that we extend our competencies to meet cases and situations that challenge our sometimes deeply held assumptions and values. When this happens, doctors need opportunities for deep reflection, as provided by the sort of supervision we are describing. As Fish and Coles (2005) say, membership of a profession brings with it the moral duty for professionals to be aware of the values (personal and professional) that drive their judgements and actions and the duty to recognize and take account of them as part of their on-the-spot responses. Using ongoing supervision is one way of understanding how behaviour, attitudes and values mirror themselves between the doctor's personal and practice life. It offers an opportunity to explore the core meaning of being a professional (Fish and Twinn 1997) as someone who 'seeks a broad understanding of their practice, paying attention not only to their developing competence, but also to the fundamental purposes and values that underpin their work' (Golby 1993).

Initially in clinical supervision, issues presented are likely to be recounted with the emphasis on the patient or clinical situation. But over time, the issues supervisees bring to supervision often deepen and reflect the issues they recognize as shaping the way they work, that of course reflect in the patient care they offer and invite a more challenging approach that looks at the supervisees' personal resonance to the issues presented. This leads to opportunities for change not only at the level of clinical practice but also at the personal level. That in turn has an impact on the culture of the teams and organizations we work in and with. Over time supervisees may address issues that at first would not have been contemplated by them.

An integrated approach

One framework that has helped one of us (David) to reflect on supervisees' needs in different supervisory settings has been to think of doctors' educational, support and development needs in three different contexts – the personal, the practice and the organizational. This framework allows the supervisee and supervisor to have a preliminary discussion about the focus of the supervision they are jointly undertaking, and to consider it in a broad context. It provides doctors with a structure to begin mapping the impact, challenges and opportunities of the accelerating healthcare reforms and increased complexity levels of reorganizations that most doctors are facing.

The educational needs link to more formal learning that is highlighted or directed in supervision, the support role may require a more caring function to explore and move through periods of challenge and uncertainty, while the development needs may include the inner change and the tranformational or reframing process that the supervisee may need to go through. Different doctors often find they identify with problems in some of the grids, but find it more difficult to talk about or see issues in others, although this may change at different stages of one's professional career. In practice, shifts in one area of the grid often provide an opportunity to explore the implications in other areas as well. As such, the 'matrix' can be a useful mapping tool for the supervisor as well as the supervisee. Table 1.1 gives examples of issues that might present but that might be different depending on whether the focus was more on educational, managerial or clinical supervision. We would encourage supervisees

Table 1.1 The supervision matrix

	Education	*Support*	*Development*
Personal	Being told new information, I might have done it differently	Being heard – I'm not alone with this	What I found hard was …; I wonder if this is why
Practice	Learning from how others work	Sharing practice problems	Reflecting on critical events
Professional/ Organizational	Establishing best practice	Knowing about professional norms and how I fit in	Looking at career path, choices and how I can contribute to my professional bodies

to reflect on and identify their needs in each area and consider especially those areas they might not immediately be attracted to, or that do not initially 'jump out at them' as difficulties in one part of the matrix are often linked to challenges in others. For example, when doctors have perceived they have made errors in their practice, they might not immediately see the link to lack of support, burn out or feeling depressed (West *et al.* 2006).

Summary

Supervision's primary purpose is sometimes taken to be to develop the supervisee at work and to ensure the welfare of patients (Carroll 1996). Different styles of supervision seek to achieve this in different ways and many supervisors will carry a mix of roles. Broadening the range of issues that can be addressed in any supervisory relationship is key to understanding why patterns of behaviour develop and are maintained. Exploring the issues more deeply, and uncovering the underlying attitudes and values that determine how we act, makes significant and sustainable change possible in our practice for our own well-being and the welfare of patients.

Supervision as we describe above, and throughout this book, explores the relationship between doctor and patient, helping to uncover hidden aspects of the supervisee (and supervisor) that represent blind spots in our clinical work. It provides a chance to understand and respond to situations in a more aware way, sometimes breaking patterns of response that have been repeated many times or that are ingrained in our behaviour. This in turn can transform how we engage with situations we previously found difficult. As one supervisee said,

> It transformed what I considered to be wounds, which I had unknowingly kept hidden, to something that was an opportunity and challenge to change, and that now is something I am happy to talk about and reveal to others like a battle scar I am proud to carry.

While recognizing that there is a legitimate fear of 'supervision for supervision's sake', we must also recognize that there is a reluctance to look at things closely in case we do not like what we see. Many doctors already work to the highest motives and we wish to support this while encouraging practices and reflection that enable us to glimpse aspects of our work from a different perspective – what we might call the 'aha' moment (Owen 2007). Often the way the supervisee and supervisor personalize and extend the way they work is reflected in the working agreement between both parties in what we call the supervisory agreement.

Clinical supervision supports doctors in coping with the variety of stressful situations that clinical practice brings, including talking about issues concerning feeling uncertain and disillusioned. While making the support of the doctor (supervisee) explicit, this is done in the knowledge that, when well supported, the doctor is more likely to be able to offer a higher level of care, to notice and respond to educational needs, and to work towards team and organizational goals.

Note

1. Hawkins and Shohet use the word client in relation to the helping profession but we think this can be interchanged with patient.

References

Burton, J. and Launer, J. (2003) *Supervision and Support in Primary Care*. Abingdon: Radcliffe.

Carroll, M. (1996) *Counselling Supervision: Theory, Skills and Practice*. London: Cassell.

Fish, D. and Coles, C. (2005) *Medical Education: Developing a Curriculum for Practice*. Maidenhead: Open University Press.

Fish, D. and Twinn, S. (1997) *Quality Clinical Supervision in the Health Care Professions*: *Principled Approaches to Practice*. Oxford: Butterworth-Heinemann.

Foster, K. (2009) Learning about medical professionalism – don't forget emotion!, *Clinical Teacher*, 6(1): 9–12.

Golby, M. (1993) Educational research: trick or treat?, *Exeter Society for Curriculum Studies*, 15(3): 5–8.

Hawkins, P. and Shohet, R. (2006) *Supervision in the Helping Professions*, 3rd edn. Maidenhead: Open University Press.

Hawkins, P. and Shohet, R. (2012) *Supervision in the Helping Professions*, 4th edn. Maidenhead: Open University Press.

Hunt, P. (1986) Supervision, *Marriage Guidance*, Spring, 15–22.

Johns, C. (1999) *Becoming a Reflective Practitioner*. Oxford: Blackwell Publishing.

Kennedy, T. (2009) Towards a tighter link between supervision and trainee ability, *Medical Education*, 43: 1126–8.

Kenny, N., Mann, K. and MacLeod, H. (2003) Role modelling in physicians' professional formation: reconsidering an essential but untapped educational strategy, *Academic Medicine*, 78(12) 1203–21.

Launer, J. (2003) Practice, supervision, consultancy and appraisal: a continuum of learning, *British Journal of General Practice*, 53: 662–5.

Launer, J. (2006) *Supervision, Mentoring and Coaching: One-to-One Learning Encounters in Medical Education*. Edinburgh: Association for the Study of Medical Education.

Lave, J. and Wenger, E. (1991) *Situated Learning: Legitimate Peripheral Participation*. Cambridge: Cambridge University Press.

Mollon, P. (1989) Anxiety, supervision and a space for thinking: some narcissistic perils for clinical psychologists in learning psychotherapy, *British Journal of Psychology*, 62: 113–22.

Nielsen, H. G. and Tulinius, C. (2009) Preventing burnout among general practitioners: is there a possible route?, *Education for Primary Care*, 20: 353–9.

Owen, D. (2007) The aha moment, in R. Shohet (ed.) *Passionate Supervision*. London: Jessica Kingsley Publishers.

Proctor, B. (2001) Training for the supervision alliance: attitude, skills and intention, in J. Cutliffe, T. Butterworth and B. Proctor (eds) *Fundamental Themes in Clinical Supervision*. London and New York: Routledge.

West, C. P., Huschka, M. M., Novotny, P. J. *et al.* (2006) Association of perceived medical errors with resident distress and empathy: a prospective longitudinal study, *Journal of the American Medical Association*, 296: 1071–8.

2   The five realms

David Owen

Editors' introduction

This chapter builds on the previous introduction. In it David Owen describes a comprehensive model of supervision, developed from his use of Hawkins and Shohet's seven-eyed model in supervision of doctors. He illustrates how the model can be used to gear supervision to the needs of the doctor, taking into account the patient, his or her illness and the broader context that shapes the medical profession. At any one time the supervisor has many options and, by taking the reader through the different realms, the author's intention is to raise awareness of these options so that the one most relevant and useful can be chosen. The five realms are a map which enables supervisor and supervisee to navigate the territory more skilfully and to see each intervention and aspect of supervision as part of an holistic approach.

Overview of chapter

In this chapter I describe a model that I have found useful when working as a supervisor with doctors. It allows supervision to focus on all aspects of, and all parties in the therapeutic relationship, namely the disease, the patient, the doctor, the supervisor and the broader context in which both care and supervision are given. I give examples of supervision and pointers for supervisees and supervisors who might want to incorporate aspects of this approach.

Introduction

In practice, supervision works on many levels of focus simultaneously and the supervision relationship is probably the single most important factor for the effectiveness of supervision.

(Kilminster and Jolly 2000)

In every clinical relationship the doctor holds an extraordinary position in relation to the patient. When, as doctors, we find ourselves in challenging situations, it often appears that the problem is due to the patient or the illness. We understandably try to 'fix it', often without really taking on board the impact of the problem on ourselves or our impact on the problem. Failing to pay attention to what is evoked in us and what we evoke in others is a major cause of patient and doctor dissatisfaction that may, in some cases, erode the well-being of both parties. This can go on and undermine the very healthcare structures upon which we rely to treat patients and support ourselves.

This chapter offers a model that I call the Five Realms, which is useful in supporting doctors to look at all aspects of the clinical relationship.

These five realms are:

1   The realm of the illness, including the diagnosis and disease management.
2   The realm of the patient, including the patient's subjective experience of the illness and the relationship of the patient to his or her family and environment.
3   The realm of the doctor, including the doctor–patient relationship, the doctor's relationship with colleagues, work and home environment, as well as the doctor's professional needs and personal well-being.
4   The realm of the supervisor, including the supervisor–doctor (supervisee) relationship.
5   The broader organizational, cultural and socio-economic context in which we practise.

This model has a simple structure that I have found fits the requirements of a wide range of doctors interested in a practical 'map' and the associated tools for extending the scope of clinical supervision. It has emerged from my training and experience of working with the 'seven-eyed model of supervision' described by Peter Hawkins and Robin Shohet (2006). The five realms model both allows the exploration of the relationship between different parties such as the doctor–patient relationship and allows the supervisor and supervisee to focus explicitly on the different aspects of care and supervision that influence a doctor's work.

Some of the benefits of working in supervision with the five realms described here is that it links together and contributes to a virtuous cycle of improvement in disease management, patient communication (and satisfaction) and doctor well-being. It also commonly enhances doctor enthusiasm and addresses professional isolation. It invites a patient–doctor relationship that is engaged and collaborative, as well as allowing doctors to process their feelings about those things they cannot change or that they find difficult to change, and exploring how to change those things that they can. In addition this model empowers doctors to look at and, if appropriate, challenge unhelpful cultural, social and professional beliefs.

Each of the five realms invites a different way of looking at an issue, giving five different perspectives to understand and explore a doctor's professional relationships. These five realms can be represented as sitting one inside the other like Russian dolls, as illustrated in Figure 2.1.

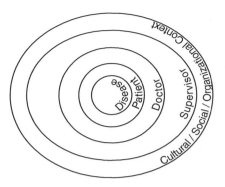

Figure 2.1   The five realms

In the realm of the disease the doctor reviews a particular patient's treatment or diagnosis. In the realm of the patient, the doctor explores the wider impact and interaction between the patient and the disease and provides an opportunity to reflect more holistically on the patient's needs. The third realm focuses on the doctor and includes the therapeutic relationship. The fourth realm looks at the relationship between the supervisor and supervisee and uses the supervisor's reaction during supervision to illuminate aspects of the supervisee and his or her work. Issues with colleagues and other members of a healthcare team or practice organization arise especially in Realms 3 and 4 as they impact on a doctor's ability to care for a patient. The fifth realm looks at the broader social, cultural and organizational contexts that influence the other four realms including the context in which illness occurs, a patient is cared for, a doctor practises and supervision takes place.

While some issues appear to focus mainly in one realm, my experience is that the five realms or perspectives do not exist independently from each other but are dynamically intertwined.

CASE EXAMPLE: DOCTOR A

In one supervision session Doctor A brought an apparently simple question about the drug of choice for a particular condition. Doctor A felt uneasy while explaining the risk–benefits of a particular drug to a patient. Exploring it further, Doctor A commented that, although the drug being recommended was the 'drug of choice', he would not take it himself if he had the same condition as the patient. This in turn led him to look at his own feelings about prescribing drugs that he personally had reservations about. Once this had been done, Doctor A was much clearer about how to explain and explore the different treatment options with his patient.

Different supervisees and supervisors will often have a personal preference about how they work, and will find the perspective offered by looking into some of these realms easier than others. In my experience, often the deepest insights and most profound changes come when supervisees are able to explore one of their less preferred ways of working. One of the most important aspects of the supervisor's role is to make help supervisees feel safe enough to see things from a different perspective and support them with looking at how they might do things differently.

In the rest of this chapter I will go on to look in more detail at the five realms, and some of the supervisory processes that can be used in each. As you read I invite you to imagine using them on an issue of your own.

Realm 1: the disease

Supervision in the realm of the disease looks in detail at diagnosis and treatment options. In some ways the patient expects to come to the doctor with symptoms of an illness and leave with the diagnosis of a disease. Most doctors already have a comprehensive palette of diagnostic labels and a tool bag of interventions, which in many situations suffice to meet the needs of the patient. When the doctor is uncertain about either diagnosis or intervention there are a number of ways that they can easily get information or support without taking part in a formal supervisory process. My experience, however, is that while many doctors are used to, and proficient in, gaining and updating this knowledge base, there are often 'blind spots' for some doctors which supervision can help identify and address. In effective supervision the supervisee and supervisor may well be able to generate a 'menu' of options to resolve an issue such as a symptom picture with no clear diagnosis or an illness with no clear treatment available.

Additionally, supervision can help in the many areas of clinical work where the non-specific care that a doctor offers is as important as any specific treatment or intervention. This 'art of medicine' often receives less attention than the 'scientific' aspects, but is equally important in terms of disease management (Helman 2004). For example, in managing long-standing chronic disease or offering palliative care the doctor will often benefit from a supportive and structured reflective space such as that offered by supervision.

Another area that supervisees often find helpful – possibly through 'role-play' – is to rehearse providing information on a diagnosis, a treatment plan or advice on lifestyle (for disease modification or prevention). It can also help to elucidate how a doctor might talk about treatments that carry frequent or serious risk of adverse effects, or when giving advice on screening for a condition. Although clarity about the information required is part of the issue, more often the challenge comes in communicating it. A simple way to invite reflection is to ask, 'If you were the patient, how would you like this communicated?', and compare this to '. . . how would you not want it communicated?'.

CASE EXAMPLE: ARATI

Arati used supervision to explore the difficulties she experienced when changing a patient from an expensive drug to a cheaper alternative while following new practice guidelines. The patient had brought the new drug back to Arati and, 'dumping it' in a tatty plastic bag on Arati's desk, reeled off a list of reasons why she wanted to be given the original more expensive one. In supervision Arati explored the pros and cons of the different treatments for the patient, how she felt about the practice guidelines and how doctors in the practice worked together. Arati, by role-playing the patient, then glimpsed how, for this patient, the exchange was less about 'the drug' positioned between the doctor and patient, and more about the patient's anxiety about her long-term management plan. In supervision Arati explored several strategies on how a transition to the new treatment might be managed and how to present these to her patient and colleagues.

Finally, the personal and financial burden placed on doctors undergoing litigation is huge. While supervision cannot offer a place to review every single treatment or diagnosis, it does help to develop what some doctors describe as a 'sixth sense' or 'intuitive alarm' about the diagnosis or treatment of a disease that need revisiting. Often the patients that supervisees first bring to supervision are the ones that have set this alarm going. Although supervised practice is becoming a common way of supporting doctors in difficulty, my experience is that supervision appears to be a very effective way of preventing doctors from getting into difficulty in the first place.

Realm 2: the patient

Clinical management involves more than an awareness of how a disease expresses itself in a patient; it also looks at each individual's susceptibility and reaction to a disease. It requires an openness to patients' preferences and an understanding of their likely response to any advice and treatment offered. The patient is frequently in an unfamiliar state, both physically and emotionally, with uncertainty about how a disease might unfold or what treatment options are available. In chronic disease, where there may be no one best treatment, these factors are increased. Supervision is a place where the impact of the disease and treatment on a patient, and issues that relate to the individual management of a patient, can be reviewed and explored. While this learning is core to much of a doctor's general and specialist training, the issues remain central to a doctor's clinical competence. For example, exploring a patient's behaviours in supervision – whether abrasive, non-compliant, destructive or 'sabotaging' – can reveal much about the person who has the illness. Another issue that often presents in supervision is the management of patients with no clear diagnosis, no clear prognosis or no obvious treatment. Kroenke and Mangelsdorff (1989) studied fourteen prevalent symptoms in ambulatory care and undertook a retrospective review of outpatient records to determine the incidence, aetiology, evaluation and outcome of the symptoms. In only 16 per cent of cases was an organic cause for the symptoms found; 10 per cent of cases were thought to be of psychological origin and in close to 75 per cent no known cause was found. In most cases, diagnostic evaluations were found to be expensive and unproductive. Such patients may consult a number of doctors, are frequently dissatisfied, and can take up a disproportionate amount of diagnostic and therapeutic resources. Supervision allows doctors to explore how they can work with their uncertainty and meaningfully assist patients with their illness despite this uncertainty. This often starts with an understanding of the psycho-social context in which the patient lives and how this is affected by the illness. While many doctors will invite patients to offer such personal information in order to 'take it into account', patients will often hold back from disclosing such information if they perceive that in some way the doctor cannot manage all the thoughts and feelings that might be evoked in them. Doctors in regular clinical supervision often report feeling greater sensitivity and openness to this information. It is as if while they are being 'held' in supervision they are more able to see the whole patient.

One of the clues that a supervisee has failed to see the patient adequately, or has not taken into account his or her personal and idiosyncratic needs is that, as a supervisor, you find yourself wondering what the patient is 'really like'. It is as if the patient being discussed is 'in grey', 'hidden' or 'masked' in some way by the medical problem or treatment, with only the smallest part of the patient being glimpsed. It is one reason why even highly competent doctors discussing the clinical management of a difficult case appear to struggle when no clear strategy or intervention 'jumps out'. When the patient has been partially 'blocked out', all you can do is fall back on previous patterns of intervention rather than explore strategies that address an individual patient's needs. One way of exploring this in a supervision session is to encourage the supervisee to describe the patient in detail using as many senses as possible. For example, he could describe what clothes the patient was wearing, or any make-up or jewellery. How did the patient walk into the consulting room; what was the expression on her face? Supervisees could recall what they heard, the exact words the patient used, any odour or the sensation if they shook hands. These all help to 'bring the patient into the room'.

CASE EXAMPLE: DOCTOR B

One supervisee, Doctor B, was left feeling anxious that a patient appeared to be fault finding and Doctor B felt she was complaining about her. When she called to mind her patient, using the exercise above, Doctor B remembered the patient had walked into the room like 'a startled sparrow' with a very precise manner, and was dressed extremely smartly and had a fastidious nature. After recalling this, Doctor B was able to recognize the patient's behaviour in the consultation as part of her general behaviour rather than it relating specifically to her medical competence. Doctor B went on to rehearse some things she might do differently, to put this patient and similar patients at ease, and at the same time noting how her own defensiveness could contribute to a patient's defensive behaviour.

In another example a supervisee presented a frequently attending patient who the doctor thought had unrealistic expectations of what could be achieved with the treatment available. In supervision the doctor explored what she might do to help the patient express his expectations and what the patient might really want but be unable to ask for. Once the doctor recognized that she could encourage the patient to talk about these without having to have all the answers, the doctor felt more empathy towards the patient. From this position the doctor found it easier to offer supportive and constructive advice and to discuss with the patient the impact on her of his frequent attendance. The doctor could see that the patient's own despair was mirrored by her own heartsink feelings. Going into Realm 3, the supervisor was able to work with the doctor's own feelings to recognize and gain further insight into how the patient felt.

Realm 3: the doctor/supervisee

Medical work is inherently imprecise and always involves personal fallibility.
(Coles 2006)

In this realm, supervisors invite supervisees to notice what is happening to them when they are with the patient. It provides an opportunity for supervisees to look at their own internal process and how this is affected by the patient–doctor relationship, which in turn influences the clinical care of the patient. It is invaluable when exploring the types of patients that trigger an almost reflex type of emotional response in the doctor (sometimes refered to as 'having our buttons pushed'), and is important when doctors unknowingly carry their own unrealistic expectations or unmet needs into a thera-peutic relationship. As the example above of the heartsink patient shows, it is often a way of projecting the doctor's difficulty on to the patient and then labelling the patient. It includes common patterns of behaviour in the doctor that can evoke unex-pected behaviour from patients and lead to inappropriate responses that can jeopardize a patient's treatment or a doctor's professional behaviour. A supervisor might notice a doctor repeating 'key' words or phrases or using particular hand movements when talking about a patient behaving in a certain way. So, for example, I might notice that a doctor sighs a lot when talking about a patient; he might bunch his fists up or become restless. Just drawing the doctor's attention to these and gently 'wondering what they mean' can often enable the doctor to glimpse aspects of the patient and their relation-ship that are otherwise invisible to them. When the doctor is able to recognize these things and look at what they mean in supervision it frequently leads to a new insight. This in turn often leads to an improvement not only in the care of the patient and other similar patients but also to the enjoyment and well-being of the doctor.

It is not unusual for doctors struggling with a particular aspect of their practice to find that the issue reoccurs. Often a 'way of coping' develops that may have an impact on the doctor's personal life, or on the organization or team in which he or she works. When supervising in this realm, tensions between doctors, colleagues and healthcare team members can sometimes surface. These may or may not be directly related to the clinical care of a particular patient. However, they can have a huge effect on a doctor's ability to care for patients and the provision of a service generally. They may surface in Realm 3 through their impact on the doctor or when reviewing Realm 5 and considering the wider context of a doctor's work. When these issues are resolved it often has a significant benefit for the doctor, her work and those working with her. So while supervision frequently focuses on one specific issue or patient, the benefits for the patient, the doctor and those who work with that doctor can be far reaching.

The late paediatrician, Donald Winnicott (1954), introduced the concept of the 'good-enough mother' – the mother who, when her child throws the food back at her, does not overreact to this as a personal attack or sink under feelings of inadequacy and guilt, but can hear this event as the child expressing its temporary inability to cope with the external world. Winnicott points out that it is hard for any mother to be 'good-enough' unless she is held and supported by either the child's father or another supportive adult. This triad of child, mother and 'other' allows for the child to be accepted, whatever it needs to express. As Hawkins and Shohet say (2006: 3), this provides a useful analogy for supervision, where 'good-enough doctors' can survive what the patient throws at them from the patient's world and what is evoked for them from their own past experience more easily while being held in a supervisory relationship. The supervisor not only supports the doctor but also provides an opportunity for insight and learning from the experience.

Often a doctor's or patient's behaviour is driven by issues below the surface of what is explicit in a consultation. Supervision provides an opportunity to explore these implicit issues and look at how they can be managed so that the doctor and patient can have a more authentic therapeutic relationship. Clues that the doctor's or patient's behaviour is driven by issues that lie below include when strong emotions (both positive and negative) are generated in the consultation, or when normal boundaries such as time or personal contact are challenged, or even broken. It is understandable that these are difficult to 'air', and for supervision to work in this realm doctors (supervisees) must feel that supervision is a safe place to reveal their deeper thoughts and feelings. Most supervisors working in this realm are familiar with the shame that doctors often feel when they talk about exploring their limitations and what they find difficult. Similarly, most supervisors working in this way report that when supervisees open up to a third party the experience can be cathartic and provide a release from the burden they are carrying left over from some consultations.

One of the techniques I use when inviting supervisees to think about an interaction with a patient that they are not happy with, is to ask them to identify where in the consultation (or interaction) they felt most stuck. Then I ask them to describe three different options of what they might have said or done differently. The first option is what they think a wise and experienced colleague might have said or done in the same situation; it might be a previous teacher, a role model or mentor. The second, what they imagine the patient really wanted to happen at that time and what they, the supervisee, might have said or done to help make this happen for the patient. The third is to think of what they would have really liked to say (or do) to the patient, regardless of how others would interpret it. I want to stress that this is not what they would actually say but to explore what was blocking an authentic communication. For the third option, supervisees will often need some encouragement to really let go of their inhibitions. For the second and third perspectives, if supervisees are struggling to come up with options they may find it easier to imagine what the easiest option is (often giving the patient what he or she wants) and what a wild (or crazy) options is (often what they fantasize about saying but feel unable to ask for). Any of these three options may put the doctor in touch with feelings including anger, attraction, sadness, etc. Finally, supervisees can rehearse any intervention informed by, but different from the three options, on the patient. The example of Sam illustrates this.

CASE EXAMPLE: SAM

Sam talked of a patient that had harassed him as he was coming out of his practice. The patient had been drinking and grabbed him by his shirt collar and demanded Sam see his child. Sam was concerned for the child but felt threatened and so asked the receptionist to call the police. Afterwards he felt humiliated and guilty about this and avoided the patient. When he was invited to explore the three options outlined above, he thought of a mentor who would have 'never got himself into the situation' but if threatened would have known exactly what to say. In the second option, Sam thought the patient really was anxious for his child and was standing up to the authority figure that Sam represented in order to get his needs met. In the third option, Sam explored how he wished he had used martial arts to restrain the patient. When encouraged, he got in touch with his anger and indignation towards the patient. After working through these options Sam 'debriefed', talking about his unrealistic expectations of himself, the idea that there was always 'a right thing to do', his own frustration with authority and his fear and vulnerability. Rehearsing how he might respond another time he commented that his sympathy for the patient had possibly sent 'the wrong signals' and he would be much clearer about his need to feel safe in order to empathize.

Sam not only explored how he might act differently another time but something he had been 'holding' in relation to the patient shifted through the supervision. I am confident that when he sees the patient again he will be freer to act differently. Finally, it brought into focus for Sam his own issues with authority. Certainly there are times when supervisees, having presented a difficult case, end up appreciating patients for the insights they offer the doctor.

Our ability to perceive others accurately is governed by the extent to which we accurately perceive ourselves. When we are blind to an aspect of ourself we will miss this aspect in others. As such, giving or receiving supervision provides an opportunity to identify and work with our 'blind spots'. As a general rule, the more resistant we are to looking at something, the greater the impact of seeing it anew. When the patient and doctor have similar (or overlapping) blind spots, the patient or doctor can mistakenly identify qualities or features of the other as their own, and the patient and/or the doctor acts in a way that is unknowingly driven by the other (Sachs and Shapiro 1976). In supervision, such behaviour, when given time and space, surfaces and the supervisee will unknowingly enact with the supervisor aspects of the behaviour between doctor and patient in a form of 'parallel enactment'. When recognized, supervisees can explore through their relationship and behaviour with the supervisor what lies behind their behaviour and relationship with the patient. It is surprising how working through such issues in supervision can dramatically shift the way a doctor manages a specific situation or condition, a patient generally or even a whole group of patients.

However, if such issues are unable to surface, be examined or become resolved, then it is not surprising that they reoccur, 'leak out' onto colleagues, family or even onto other patients. Over time, commonly enacted behaviour can become embedded as simply the 'normal' behaviour of individuals, teams and even stereotypes of professional subgroups.

If a supervisee is struggling to identify what is being acted out in the relationship between himself and the patient, then one exercise described by Hawkins and Shohet (2006) that I find helpful is to invite the supervisee to imagine removing all exterior distractions and to intensify the imagined relationship. For example, I might ask him to imagine himself alone with a patient on a desert island and describe how we imagine they might interact. You might like to try this out for yourself, thinking of a colleague or patient with whom you feel stuck and then imagine being alone with that person. The intensity of the exercise can be increased by asking yourself to imagine that you are alone with just this person for several months (or even a few years) and to reflect on what you imagine taking place. This exercise can also help when the relationship between supervisor and supervisee seems to be fixed or stuck around a particular issue. As a supervisor I might explore with the supervisee how we might both behave differently in a different setting or if other, actual or imagined restraints were removed.

Another way to explore the realm of the supervisee is to invite her to reflect about who the others in the narrative, such as a patient, remind her of? It is not uncommon to discover that those patients we find it hardest to communicate and interact with clearly and 'cleanly' often remind us of a relative (parent, sibling or child) or 'significant other'. For some supervisees who have had experience reviewing videos of their own consultations, it can be helpful to enquire what might stand out, or what they would be embarrassed about if I were to watch a video of the interaction. Prompts might include questions like, 'What would it look like to someone else?', 'How would you feel watching someone else in this situation?', and 'What would you think was happening if it were someone else in the same situation?'

Realm 4: the supervisor

This realm focuses on supervisors' own internal awareness of themselves and how they are affected by the supervisee. It asks of supervisors that they be very present to their internal states – these could be feelings, body sensations, images which they might normally not bring into awareness. As such it is a very different focus from the preceding realms, as it invites the possibility that the problem being presented is being re-enacted in some way in the room.

Working in this fourth realm allows the supervisee and supervisor to look at what is happening in the session *as it is taking place*, in the 'here and now'. When there are unresolved issues from the past, in what we might refer to as the 'there and then', these may influence what takes place in the 'here and now'. Realm 4 can explore what happens in the supervision (and to the supervisor) that is clouded by the past. For example, in a recent supervision session I noticed I was irritated by the supervisee (here and now). As this is uncharacteristic for me I used this to wonder and explore if the supervisee was irritated by his patient. When I explored this with the supervisee he was able to acknowledge this. As is often observed in what is sometimes referred to as 'parallel process', the issue happening in the here and now of supervision mirrored the issues in the there and then of the supervisee's relationship with the patient.

Sometimes the physical sensations and feelings supervisors have during supervision reflect emotional feelings that are difficult to name, like irritation. Supervisors may use these somatic feelings to guide their work and observe or enquire about similar movements, body language or somatic feelings in the supervisee based on what they are picking up in the here and now. So they might say something like, 'I notice I am becoming a bit restless and am feeling slightly anxious right now and I wonder if this is how you feel with your patient or how your patient might feel?' An intervention like this uses the somatic sensation and the emotional feeling in the here and now as a possible mirror of the supervisee/patient relationship. The following example illustrates how supervisors can use their own emotional awareness to explore the supervisee and patient relationship.

CASE EXAMPLE: SUE

In a supervision session with a general practitioner, let us call her Sue, we were exploring the case of a patient that had committed suicide. The patient was in her early twenties with a young child and the GP had been supporting her over a number of years. Sue had not been available to speak to the patient shortly before she committed suicide and the patient had instead spoken to another doctor in the practice. When the practice found out about the suicide Sue was left a short message that she picked up at the beginning of her surgery. Sue was wanting to address how the practice communicated such events and was working things through in quite a detached way. In supervision Sue suggested several ideas for how things could be fixed but would quickly go on to explain why these were impractical. As the supervisor I became quite aware of how inappropriately withdrawn I was feeling during the hunt for a solution to the communication problems. I tentatively explained how I was feeling and asked Sue if she recognized feeling withdrawn in any aspect of the management of the patient. Sue was surprised at first and said she felt disappointed with me for withdrawing. I explained I was not withdrawing but noticing and reporting to her how I felt. I recognized it was atypical for me to feel withdrawn in such a situation and so wanted her to think about where these feelings might be coming from. (Often an intial defence or denial can affirm that the supervisor is exploring something of importance.) Sue started to speak about how she felt about the other doctor in the practice who has seen the patient. She was disappointed the other doctor had not spoken to her about the patient. She spoke about feeling guilty about what had happened. When I asked her to speak more about this she described feeling overwhelmed about the plight of the patient and the aloneness of the child. Asked if these feelings reminded her of how she had felt in the past (moving into Realm 3), Sue spoke about feeling alone at times as a child and realized she had felt maternal towards the patient. Sue became tearful talking about how it must have been awful for the patient feeling so alone and now the baby being alone. After exploring this Sue went on to talk about how she recognized that by focusing on how the doctors communicated at the practice she was, in a way, withrawing from the distress she felt. Once Sue had recognized this she was both able to work through her feelings towards the patient and her upset at her patient's death and think about how to raise it with partners as a significant event at the next practitioners' meeting.

The emotional awareness of the supervisor is an important resource, especially, I find, when navigating in more uncertain or 'stuck' cases. There are many other examples of how supervisors can use what they notice about themselves and their behaviour in supervision. This may include supervisors noticing their own posture, 'body language' or where they are sitting in relationship to the supervisee. So, for example, if I notice I am sitting in a closed or defensive posture I may explore if there is defensiveness in the supervisee and/or patient. If I find I am not attending to time boundaries or fail to be explicit about contracting, I might explore in what way these issues might be mirrored in the supervisee's issues. While it is not always necessary to articulate to the supervisee what is being noticed by the supervisor in Realm 4, I have found it a way to open up a dialogue about what might otherwise be masked or hidden to the supervisee. Indeed, it often appears to me that the more difficult it is for a supervisee to get in touch with a feeling, behaviour or issue in supervision the more these are seemingly unconsciously broadcast by the supervisee for the supervisor to 'tune into'.

Realm 5: the broader context

Paradoxically the status and rewards of being a doctor may well be part of society's compensation for what doctors are expected to carry and the price they pay in relation to their well being.

(Wallace *et al.* 2009)

Realm 5 is qualitatively different from the other realms in that it explores the organizational, social and cultural context of each of the other realms. As a supervisor, I frequently invite a supervisee to explore this as a pragmatic check on what is realistic in the situation, what I sometimes refer to as a 'reality check'. I may do this while working in any realm or as part of bringing together the different insights from supervision into an appropriate plan of action. In the earlier example of Arati working with a patient whose medication was changed due to the financial restraints, it was quite appropriate to check out if Arati agreed with this guideline from her general practice. Working in this realm often includes reflecting on how the insights of supervisees can be shared with those they work with, the professional resources available to the patient and the availability of personal and professional support to the supervisees. Considering the broader context often offers three additional benefits. It encourages a less isolated and more integrated view of an individual's work. It can empower supervisees to inter-act with and influence the organizations and teams with which they work. It allows supervisees to look at what other personal and professional support is available to them and to those they work with.

One example of how patients, doctors, teams and organizations are interlinked is illustrated through the issue of time management. It seems most doctors could bring some aspect of this to supervision. It can present as a patient over-running his or her allotted appointment time, a doctor running late for appointments, long waiting lists, or some frustration with how long something takes to happen.

CASE EXAMPLE

One supervisee noticed that even right after a break, or at the beginning of a clinic, they would still be late starting. This created stress for patients, doctors and practice staff and it came to a head one day when a patient arrived late for an appointment because he assumed the clinic would run late. Exploring this in supervision revealed that behind the reality of frequent short appointments, the doctor felt that there was never enough time and that even if they ever did run to time at work, extra patients would then be 'fitted in', so making them finish late anyway. On deeper reflection, the supervisee realized that by running late they had a sense of some control and power over their appointment list. The supervision session went on to look at how the supervisee could work with other team members to address the way extra patients were distributed. At a later session the supervisee reported they had improved their running to time and that, following a team discussion, staff had a clearer sense of 'what was expected and when'.

Often the techniques used in one realm can be extended to work in other realms. For example, working with role-play to look at an issue can be extended to explore an organizational element by looking at how other individuals or teams that might influence the scenario can be represented. The dynamic between these different parties can often be explored more explicitly in this way.

Each individual struggling with any aspect of his or her practice provides an opportunity for the profession as a whole to engage in an honest dialogue about the nature of professional practice. In reality most often the needs of the supervisee are more immediate than this (Lake 2009) and are therefore more often the focus. However, the potential benefits for the profession as a whole and patient care generally are often commented on by those who regularly take part in this style of supervision. While professional bodies frequently encourage supervision, the reality is that it is still a long way from becoming enshrined in the normal working pattern and from becoming not just a notional requirement, but an actively sought after and integrated part of a medical professional's life. However, it is important to recognize that the provision and uptake of supervision is intertwined with cultural and organizational attitudes to talking openly about difficult things, and the way we individually and collectively respond to issues that challenge us. Often clinical supervision takes place alongside and in parallel with educational and/or management supervision. This can present a creative tension between the 'encouraging and supporting' emphasis of clinical super-vision, the 'training and assessing' of educative supervision and the 'controlling and regulating' of management supervision (see Chapter 1). We look at how the provision of supervision is subject to personal, professional and cultural influences in Chapter 12, 'Listening to resistance'.

Using the five realms in supervision

In a supervision session I might start in any of the realms but often for those new to supervision it is easier to see the relevance to the patient when beginning with the illness. I use it as a map to help supervisees recognize where they are now and where they might go to next. It describes the terrain rather than the journey itself, a menu rather than a meal. Issues that emerge in one realm frequently (not surprisingly) mirror issues that occur in others and so a supervision session will naturally flow through the different realms.

Agreeing between supervisee and supervisor on how they will work is, I find, helped by giving an overview of the five realms and discussing the relevance of each. Different supervisees at different stages of their professional life and in different practice settings may have a preference for working more in some realms than others. Similarly, there will be times when there is only enough supervisory time to focus on one realm and other times when the impact on each of the realms can be explored. This will be determined by a number of factors including whether the supervision is a one-off or a short series of sessions in response to an event, or if it forms part of a medium- or long-term arrangement when the supervisee might look at 'what has surfaced' over a period of time. While these are not mutually exclusive, there is a balance between sorting things out when they go wrong and building insight and resilience so that problems can be prevented and contained. The five realms are equally useful whether working with individuals or groups. One of the benefits of group supervision is that in some ways the group becomes the supervisor of whoever is talking (see Chapter 3). The group can monitor and feed back their observations and feelings, thus reflecting the range of responses different people may have. For example, each person may focus on one of the realms so that they are each 'in the room' at the same time and can feed back from that perspective. In all cases it is important to balance the support on offer, without the supervisor and supervisee colluding with each other, and the amount of challenge, without the judgement and criticism that sometimes greets doctors who are prepared to talk about what they find difficult. As Thornton (2010) points out in her chapter on supervision groups, it is helpful if the group supervisor is aware of the importance of group dynamics so that he or she can point out when a group or group member is identifying with, or projecting, a role onto others.

This same supervisory approach can be equally helpful when working through issues with colleagues. When a supervisee chooses to look at an issue with a colleague then the same five realms can be used – the realm of the patient being exchanged for the realm of the colleague with whom there is an issue, and the realm of the illness replaced by 'the problem'.

Summary

The purpose of this chapter has been to look at the five realms of supervision, and how having this map benefits supervision. I hope it is clear that our relationship with our colleagues, the teams we work in and our practice and professional organizations can also benefit, and that the supervisor may also learn and develop personally during this process. Just as in clinical practice, as we get more competent more difficult issues present, so in supervision as we develop we are likely to attract and reveal more deep-seated issues and this helps us to work more in the realms with which we are less familiar.

Many doctors can recall experiences in their early medical career where they felt it best not to talk about the things they found difficult or mistakes they may have made for fear of being blamed, criticized, humiliated, or judged harshly. It is therefore not surprising that some go through their career finding it difficult to talk about issues they find challenging. Using the five realms provides a model not just for sustaining the provision of high-quality care to patients but, equally importantly, for developing the insight and resilience of the supervisee. While we, as doctors, must focus intently on some aspects of a patient's needs, it is inevitable that other aspects of the patient will be hidden or unclear. Using the model of the five realms can help as a way of exploring these aspects in situations where we have to look a bit deeper. The model helps provide a structure with which we can face our limitations, sit with uncertainty, and explore the unknown. It is not a question of training to reach a point where we might be all things to all patients; rather it is recognizing that at all times we will encounter situations that challenge us, and that when we need support, airing what would otherwise remain hidden is an essential part of maintaining the care we give and our own well-being.

For those new to the type of clinical supervision described in this book I would like to think the idea of the five realms will encourage you to explore 'new territories'. Aspects of this model can be combined with other models offered elsewhere. Indeed I encourage you to personalize it and, as my supervisors have encouraged me, to 'make it your own'. I hope that this chapter has introduced you to new ways of working while both consolidating what you already use and also enabling you to develop and extend your own individual approach to supervising and being supervised.

Acknowledgements

This chapter has built on chapter 7 of Hawkins and Shohet (2006). Their model is relevant for all professions, but in the case examples and particularly focusing on the realm of the illness, I have adapted it to make it relevant for doctors.

References

Coles, C. (2006) Uncertainty in a world of regulation, *Advances in Psychiatric Treatment*, 12: 397–403.

Hawkins, P. and Shohet, R. (2006) *Supervision in the Helping Professions*. Maidenhead: Open University Press.

Helman, C. (2004) *Suburban Shaman.* London: Hammersmith Press.

Kilminster, S. M. and Jolly, B. C. (2000) Effective supervision in clinical practice settings: a literature review, *Medical Education*, 34: 827–40.

Kroenke, K. and Mangelsdorff, A. D. (1989) Common symptoms in ambulatory care: incidence, evaluation, therapy, and outcome, *American Journal of Medicine*, 86: 262–6.

Lake, J. (2009) Doctors in difficulty and revalidation: where next for the medical profession?, *Medical Education*, 43: 611–12.

Sachs, D. M. and Shapiro, S. H. (1976) On parallel processes in therapy and teaching, *Psychoanalytic Quarterly*, 45: 394–415.

Thornton, C. (2010) Supervision groups, in *Group and Team Coaching: The Essential Guide.* London: Routledge.

Wallace, J., Lemaire, J. and Ghali, W. (2009) Physical wellness: a missing quality indicator, *Lancet*, 374: 1714–21.

Winnicott, D. (1954) Mind and its relation to the psyche-soma, *British Journal of Medical Psychology,* 27: 201–9.

3　The Balint group as a form of supervision

Paul Sackin and John Salinsky

Editors' introduction

We spent a lot of time deliberating the order of chapters in this book. In placing this chapter here we wanted both to honour the Balint group as perhaps the oldest consistent attempt to introduce reflective practice into the medical profession and to present the important principles embodied in this approach. As the authors write, the group acts as the supervisor. We think that this approach, which when done well empowers all participants, serves as an example of how supervisor and supervisees can combine with minimum input from the leader who acts as a guide rather than expert. In this way, although it is a form of group supervision, its philosophy is relevant to individual supervision.

Overview of chapter

In this chapter we will discuss the role of Balint groups for doctors and other health professionals. We will outline the history of these groups, describing Michael Balint's original aims for the groups and how they have developed in the sixty years since they started. We will then take a vignette from a 'typical' group and discuss what went on. Finally we will offer a 'question and answer' section that we hope will clarify the role of Balint groups in supervision.

For those not familiar with Balint groups our chapter will serve as a useful introduction to the method and maybe dispel some of the myths about this approach. The difference from most other methods described in the book is that the group acts as the 'supervisor'; the leader guides the group but does not directly 'supervise' the presenting doctor.

The beginning of Balint groups

The Balint group may well be one of the earliest forms of supervision for family doctors. The group and the method are named after Michael Balint who was a physician and psychoanalyst born in Budapest, Hungary in 1896. Balint emigrated to England in the 1930s to escape from the Nazi occupation of Eastern Europe and in 1948 he joined the staff of the Tavistock Clinic in London.

In the early 1950s Michael and his wife, Enid Balint, began holding regular seminars for general practitioners. The declared aim was to help general practitioners (GPs) towards a better understanding of what Balint called 'the psychological aspect of general practice'. Morale in general practice was very low at the time. One of the effects of the new National Health Service had been to make the GPs feel even more inferior to their consultant colleagues. The hospitals seemed to have the monopoly of high-technology scientific medicine, which was able to diagnose and treat serious illnesses with increasing success. Meanwhile, the GPs had to cope with an overwhelming number of patients whose symptoms seemed to make no sense and for which there was no diagnosis in the textbooks. Many patients were also depressed and anxious. GPs in London who were psychologically minded suspected that emotional factors might be important and were eager to learn more. But what Balint had to offer was not quite what they had expected. They found that the seminars were based on case discussion rather than the didactic teaching to which they were accustomed. It was disconcerting at first; yet for many of the early group members, it was a revelation.

Michael's father had been a GP and he always felt that the value of the GP's work was not given the respect it deserved. He described the process of the seminars as a 'research-cum-training', indicating that an important part of their purpose was to examine what actually went on in general practice. He felt that the most powerful 'drug' that GPs had at their disposal was their own relationship with the patient. But like any drug it could be harmful if its 'pharmacology' was not properly understood.

The work of the early groups was described in Balint's book *The Doctor, his Patient and the Illness* (Balint 1957). This became one of the key texts in the renaissance of general practice all over the world.

Learning to listen

The seminars consisted of a group of eight to ten GPs with Michael acting as group leader or facilitator. Later groups were led by Michael and Enid jointly. The doctors were invited to talk about patients who were troubling them. They were asked not to use notes because Michael felt that this would greatly enhance spontaneity and free association. After the presentation had been heard without interruption, the group would discuss the case under the guidance of the group leaders. What did this guidance consist of? Balint believed that the doctors needed, first of all, to learn to listen to their patients in a new kind of way. To begin with, they were expected to invite the patient back for a 'long interview' of up to an hour. This was an entirely new idea for most GPs and its results were sensational. The patients relaxed and talked about their lives as well as their symptoms. Painful stories from the past could be told for the first time. The doctor would realize how important he or she was in the patient's life. Even if the physical symptoms persisted, the fact that doctor and patient were more in touch with each other emotionally made the relationship productive. Some doctors repeated the long interview and embarked on a kind of GP psychotherapy. Others were concerned that by giving so much time to a selected few they were neglecting the equally pressing needs of their other patients. Balint thought about this and then decided to switch the emphasis to what went on in the ordinary five- or ten-minute consultation. This change of direction was described in the book *Six Minutes for the Patient* (Balint and Norell 1973). Once the patient was recognized as a person with human feelings, not so different from those of the doctor, it was possible to achieve considerable progress in a relatively short consultation, especially if it was repeated at intervals of a week or two. We must remember that there were no books on the consultation and no teaching of communication skills for doctors at the time.

The spread of Balint's influence

By the 1960s, vocational training was becoming established in the UK and Balint's ideas were widely discussed. The consultation and the doctor–patient relationship were by now seen as key elements in enabling GPs to be effective doctors for their patients. However, relatively few doctors had the opportunity to take part in a Balint group. Balint and his colleagues believed that the groups needed a psychoanalyst as a leader and there were not many analysts outside London. Some of the new vocational training schemes did incorporate Balint groups in their half-day release courses and some form of group discussion continues to be an important element of most training schemes. Meanwhile, Balint's book was translated into many languages and Balint groups were formed in other European countries, notably in Germany, France, Belgium, Holland, Scandinavia and Eastern Europe. After Balint's death, interest was maintained by the formation of Balint Societies in the UK and elsewhere. More recently, since the founding of the American Balint Society in 1990, there has been a widespread growth of Balint group teaching in family practice residency training.

Balint groups today

In the UK today there are only a few ongoing groups for established doctors. There is more activity in GP training programmes, a number of which include a Balint group as part of their half-day or day release programme. The Balint Society holds four annual courses in which doctors and psychotherapists can have the experience of taking part in a group over a day or a weekend. Training in group leading is also offered and there are some groups for students at several London teaching hospitals. There is considerable potential for more widespread use of the modern Balint group as a form of supervision at all levels of experience. We discuss later why these groups are not overly popular in the UK.

What has changed?

Balint groups in the UK today are different in a number of ways from the original model. The leaders are no longer likely to be psychoanalysts. Most groups are led by one or two GPs or a combination of a GP and a psychologist or psychotherapist. The Balint Society recommends that all group leaders have had appropriate training and accreditation. The influence of psychoanalysis is less apparent but still important. Group members may observe that their attitude to a particular patient may have been conditioned by previous experiences or personal prejudices of which they are not at first aware.

What happens in a Balint group?

The group usually consists of about eight to ten members with one or two group leaders. The group will meet regularly, usually fortnightly, for probably an hour and a half. This provides time for two presentations, one of which may be a follow-up. Follow-ups are important because they give the group the opportunity to hear about how the previous discussion has influenced the presenting doctor's relationship with the patient and whether this has been helpful.

When a group has its first meeting it is usual for the leaders and the group to agree on some basic ground rules. These will be much the same as those for all small-group activities, that is:

- Everything said within the group should be treated as confidential, whether it is about patients, colleagues or group members themselves.
- Everyone should be listened to and everyone's contribution should be respected.
- Although members may wish to talk about themselves if it seems relevant, there will be no uninvited or intrusive questioning of group members about their personal history.

The role of the group leader

The leader has to make sure that the ground rules are respected. He or she is responsible for time keeping, and has to keep an eye on the welfare of all the group members as the discussion proceeds. Someone may be trying unsuccessfully to be heard and will need to be given space. Someone else may be talking too much and may need to be reminded that, while it is good to talk, it is also good to listen. The leader has to protect group members from unwelcome interrogation or aggressive criticism. It is vital for the members to feel that the group is a safe place in which to talk about how they feel and how they have performed, without being belittled or treated harshly.

Most leaders prefer to work with a partner. This enables them to share the responsibility and to review the progress of the group together. Their status is equal unless one of the leaders is being trained by the other. If they come from different disciplines, such as general practice and psychotherapy or counselling, this is an advantage.

The presentation

When the group session begins, the leader asks who has a patient they would like to talk about. There is usually time for discussion of two patients, including follow-ups. During the presentation, the leader will listen attentively, providing a model for everyone else. At the same time he or she will be observing the mood, tone of voice and body language of the narrator to get an idea of how talking about the patient is affecting the doctors emotionally. Some presentations are quite flat in tone, perhaps reflecting the mood of a depressed patient; others are full of animation and may include direct quotations from the patient. Some express the doctor's feelings of anxiety. All these emotions are easily caught by the group members who begin to experience them too.

What sort of stories are presented in Balint groups? Typical problems include:

- the patient with chronic, medically unexplained symptoms;
- patients with what seem to be unreasonable and inappropriate demands for prescriptions, certificates, letters to excuse antisocial behaviour and referrals to specialists;
- patients who make doctors feel humiliated by referring to their lack of experience;
- depressed patients who hint at suicidal behaviour;
- difficulties in understanding people from another culture;
- complex dysfunctional families in which doctors feel trapped;
- patients who remind doctors of an aspect of themselves of which they feel ashamed.

The discussion

When the presentation has finished the presenter is thanked and the other group members are invited to have their say. There may be a lot of questioning of the presenter to begin with and some leaders try to avoid this by restricting questions to matters of fact, such as how old is the patient? What does she look like? Has she any children?

The group functions better if, at this stage, the presenter is spared questions about his own feelings with regard to the patient or why he did certain things – or what he intends to do next. This may seem strange to those who are more used to a different style of supervision, but there is a reason for it. Too much questioning of the presenter prevents the other group members from exploring and reflecting on their own thoughts about the story they have heard and the feelings it has induced in them. They need to wonder, to themselves and out loud, how the patient is feeling, what she really wants from the doctor, how they would feel if they were in the doctor's shoes.

The 'push back' phase

In order to avoid interrogation of the presenter the leader using this method will ask for an end to questions after a few minutes. He or she will then ask the presenter to move his or her chair back a few symbolic inches and then, while continuing to listen, to take no further active part in the discussion for a while. This is sometimes called the 'push back' phase. During this time group members are asked not to direct questions or statements specifically to the presenter. The group members soon get the idea of this 'game' and are usually happy to go along with it. They are now free to get to work on the case themselves using their experience, their imagination and, most importantly, their own emotional reactions. After an appropriate time (usually about twenty minutes) the presenter is invited to rejoin the group and share his or her thoughts.

To begin with, the discussion is often quite medical. The group may try to reach a physical or psychiatric diagnosis. They may suggest referral to a consultant or to a counsellor. If the patient is making worrying demands on the presenter the group may try to protect him or her by recommending strict limits on prescribing, issuing of certificates or frequency of consultation. There may be a tendency to generalize, and talk about 'patients of this kind'. Group members may introduce similar patients of their own so that the original patient is abandoned. In this situation, the group leader has to decide how long to let the discussion go on in this way before intervening. Everyone has to be allowed to have their say and express their concerns, but sooner or later, the focus has to come back to 'the patient as a person' and the emotional interaction between one doctor and one patient. Otherwise, although the discussion may be fruitful, the specific benefits of the Balint process will be lost.

The group leader's interventions

If the group is concentrating on the doctor–patient relationship the leader may need to do very little apart from monitoring the discussion and, if it seems to be drifting off course, gently steering it back. He or she will use open questions, addressed to the group as a whole rather than to individuals. The question can be turned into a statement such as: 'I wonder how the patient was feeling at the end of that consultation . . .'.

The leader might also ask (or wonder) how group members are feeling about the patient: do they like her, feel sorry for, feel angry with her or feel indifferent? What does the patient want from this doctor? What sort of doctor does she want him to be? It is customary to avoid technical terms such as 'projection' or 'transference'. But the aim is to encourage the group members to be aware of their own feelings and to experience some empathy.

If the emotional engagement with a single patient is too uncomfortable, the discussion may tend to head for calmer waters. A group member may try to reassure the presenter with a generalization such as: 'Patients with a personality disorder are untreatable; there is nothing you can do.' She may be advised to refer the patient to a specialist agency and minimize her own involvement. The leader might then intervene to say that specialist advice would indeed be helpful, but the patient will continue to need a GP and the role of the group is to try to understand what is going on in the current doctor–patient relationship.

If the group is really in danger of deserting the presented patient, the leader may bring her back into the discussion by speaking on her behalf: 'If I were that patient I would be feeling very lost and abandoned: I would feel there was nobody to take care of me...'.

In general, leader interventions have the aim of encouraging the group to stay with their feelings and to risk a little empathy with the patient. The leader will invite speculation about, and reflection on, the patient's relationships and her inner world, and will try to help them, by example, to tolerate uncertainty, ambiguity and periods of silence.

Arguably the group and the leader are working together to provide supervision. Many of the leader's interventions are analogous to the seven modes used in the process model of supervision suggested by Hawkins and Shohet (2000). Thus in mode 1, content, the therapist is encouraged to describe the client. Actually getting a picture of how the client looks, speaks, etc. can be enormously helpful in understanding the doctor–patient relationship. In mode 2 the supervisor encourages the therapist to look at the interventions he or she made with the client, while in mode 3 – perhaps the most pertinent for Balint groups – the emphasis is on the therapy relationship. Later modes look at the therapist's process, the supervisor's own process and the wider context. This last has arguably been less considered by Balint groups (Pinder *et al*. 2006), perhaps for fear that the group will digress from the main focus on the doctor–patient relationship.

In mode 5 the focus is on the supervisory relationship. 'The relationship between client and therapist are uncovered through how they are reflected in the relationship between therapist and supervisor' (Hawkins and Shohet 2000). This 'parallel process' is a key feature of Balint groups where a frequent intervention of the leader(s) is to encourage group members to look at the group process for clues as to what is happening between doctor and patient.

How does a Balint session end?

Because we are not seeking solutions, the end is often inconclusive. Leaders will not as a rule summarize the discussion or make any statement about what has been achieved. They will not make any recommendations for further management of this or any similar case. They will usually thank presenters for providing the case and ask them to give a follow-up report when they feel ready to do so. Such a way of ending may be frustrating at first for participants looking for quick solutions but ultimately it acknowledges their strengths and their ability to cope with uncertainty.

What is it like to be in a Balint group?

Let us imagine that we are taking part in a Balint group. There are nine of us, including the leader and we are sitting in a circle. Our leader is a GP who has had a lot of experience in Balint groups. Her name is Janet.

CASE EXAMPLE: JANET

'OK,' says Janet, when everyone has settled: 'Who has a patient to tell us about?'
     After a pause, Sue says, 'I have one who's been worrying me.'
     'Anybody else?' asks Janet, looking round at us all. No one else seems to have an offer at present. We are all gazing expectantly at Sue.

Sue presents her patient

So Sue begins her story. 'This is about an elderly woman who is driving me mad. I know her and her family very well, ever since I was a registrar in the practice. Her daughter and grandson were sadly killed in a car crash quite a long time ago, but she's never got over it. And yet she doesn't want to talk about it. She lives in a big house in a country area and her passion used to be horses. She still owns two horses but she isn't fit enough to look after them any more. She has had two MIs [myocardial infarctions] and she used to smoke so there's an element of COPD [chronic obstructive pulmonary disease] as well. But she is so difficult to treat and whenever anything goes wrong, which it frequently does, it's my fault. Like she gets side effects from the medication and blames me. She stopped going to cardiac rehabilitation because there was a mix-up with the transport which was apparently my fault. She expects to have home visits, which is not unreasonable, but if I say I can't go, she tries to make me feel I'm being negligent. I'm beginning to hate her! And yet I'm sorry for her and I wish she could talk about her bereavement at least a bit.

The group discussion

'Thanks, Sue,' says Janet. 'Does anyone have any questions for clarification? Is there anything more we need to know about the patient?' There are some questions about how old she is (82) and how long ago the accident was (five years ago). There's another question about whether a practice nurse could take her over, and Sue explains at some length how this was tried and didn't work. Then, Janet says, 'I think we should ask Sue to push her chair back now and just listen, while we discuss the case. (Sue moves her chair back a few inches.)

Discussion

David says she has obviously never dealt with her grief and this is why she can't make any progress. Why not refer her to a bereavement counsellor? Sarah says she wouldn't go, would she, and other people agree. Mark says it's not fair that she should behave so badly to Sue who is doing everything possible to help her. She is really lucky to have such a concerned doctor. Robert says he wonders why Sue needs to go on seeing her. Does she ever see any of the other partners, or why not send the trainee for a learning experience? (laughter). There are several other suggestions for relieving Sue of the burden. Then Janet, the group leader, says, do we think that maybe Sue wants to go on being her doctor even though the old lady gives her a hard time? What is really going on between these two? Sarah says it sounds as though Sue has replaced the daughter who was lost in the car crash and it's a sort of love–hate relationship. Without much evidence of love, says Robert. David says, she can't cry over her lost daughter and grandson, she can only be angry and Sue is the target. There is more discussion along these lines.

Then, Janet asks Sue if she would like to come back in. Sue says she found it very interesting listening to the discussion. She used to like the old lady when she was more engaged with life and was less difficult. If only she would sell that terrible old house and get a flat in town where she can see her old friends, she says. Sarah says, now you do sound like a daughter! There is more laughter and Sue joins in. But, says Janet, in fact you are not her daughter, you are her doctor. Anne, who has been quiet so far, says maybe you should detach yourself a bit from the daughter role so you don't take all this rubbish personally. Sue says, yes, I guess you are right. I certainly shouldn't be losing sleep over her. People ask if she is prepared to go on. Sue says, I'll let you know!

Comments

Of course this is a very condensed account, but hopefully it gives you some idea of the atmosphere of a typical Balint group. Note that Janet, the leader, intervenes to bring the focus back to the individual patient and her doctor. Without saying much, she helps the group to realize that there is a difference between being aware of daughter-like feelings induced by the patient, and trying to be a real daughter.

Frequently asked questions

Let us end this chapter with some questions and discussion about the role of Balint groups in supervision.

What aspects of supervision do Balint groups offer?

This book describes many aspects of supervision. These include support, burnout prevention, mentoring, encouraging reflection on one's work and discussion of the work environment. If Balint groups are to be regarded as a form of supervision, they clearly need to offer some of these features. The presentation of a 'case' for discussion provides everyone in the group with an opportunity to reflect on their own work as well as that of the presenter. This group self-reflection is facilitated by an experienced leader.

An interview study of Balint group participants (Kjeldman and Holmström 2008) suggested that participation helped them 'to endure in their job and find joy and challenge in their relationships with patients'. The groups might thus 'help GPs handle a demanding work life and prevent burnout'. A study by its participants of a remarkable Balint group that has so far been running for twenty-five years concluded that, through the group, 'our work [with patients] becomes enchanted again' (Salamon 2009). That must be a recipe for avoiding burnout!

Salamon (2009) describes how, in the group, 'we tell stories and we experience the goodness and kindness of our listeners'. In this way a Balint group is supportive. However, support is not the primary aim of a Balint group. This is to examine the doctor–patient relationship and 'increase understanding of the patient's problems, not to find solutions' (Campkin 1986). But the way these tasks are carried out should undoubtedly be supportive. As can be seen from the vignette above, presenters are not interrogated but given some protection and it is the other group members who might be challenged. In 1994 the Balint Society Council published a statement, 'What is a Balint group?' (Council of the Balint Society 1994). One of its paragraphs stated that 'the leader must above all ensure that group members, particularly the presenter, are not unduly hurt'. It went on to add that 'some increase in anxiety . . . is an almost inevitable concomitant of learning'. Working to get this balance of support and challenge, and to provide a safe environment, are key aspects of the role of a Balint group leader (as they probably are for most small group leaders) and this is one of the reasons why there is a strong move towards the accreditation of Balint leaders (Council of the Balint Society 2009).

Discussion of the work environment is another aspect of supervision. Issues related to this may well feature in a Balint group discussion anyway; they may be relevant to the doctor–patient relationship. However, there have been attempts to use the Balint method to discuss other relationships, such as those between colleagues (S. Seigel, personal communication), and it appears to work extremely well. Groups for other professional groups, such as clergy, have also been found to work well (Bryant 2007).

Why is Balint work not for all?

While we regard Balint groups as an extremely effective method of supervision, we have to accept that they are not for everybody. As we have discussed elsewhere (Salinsky and Sackin 2000), doctors (and other health workers) need defences in order to survive the hurly burly of practice life. Although Balint groups are emphatically not about breaking down these defences, some would-be participants worry that they might be. We cannot deny that to get the most out of a Balint group, participants need to have the courage to present their work and to reflect on the discussion afterwards. This may not always be a comfortable experience.

Cultural issues also play a part in limiting the acceptability of Balint work. As we have mentioned already, there is a lack of psychotherapy tradition in the UK compared with other countries, such as Germany, where the Balint movement is much stronger. In today's multiethnic world, the values of such an individually centred approach as Balint have been questioned (Pinder *et al.* 2006).

Another difficulty often voiced about Balint groups is that they are time-consuming. Certainly it will take a while to achieve the 'limited though considerable change in personality' that Michael Balint regarded as fundamental (Balint 1957). But so it would with any form of supervision. There is little doubt that smaller gains can be made on a shorter timescale. For example, Michael Balint ran a group for medical students in the 1960s (Balint *et al.* 1969) and concluded that

The 'patient-centred' approach allows the student to discern an intelligible pattern in the patient's life history and behind his physical complaints and helps him to a more reliable understanding of the patient and his illnesses.

The modern successors of this group are proving similarly effective and extremely popular with the students (Shoenberg and Suckling 2004).

Why are Balint groups not more popular?

Balint groups encountered unease and distrust from a significant number of GPs from the beginning. In our view, this was largely due to their close association with psychoanalysis, itself distrusted by many doctors. It was felt that Balint and his fellow analysts were so eager to search for psychological reasons for the patients' symptoms that group members would neglect to consider serious organic illnesses. Some doctors thought that psychoanalyst group leaders would attribute every sore throat to frustrated sexual desire and end up upsetting their patients and making fools of themselves. These days, groups in the UK are more likely to be led by a GP or a combination of a GP and a counsellor or psychotherapist and, although fantasies are encouraged in order to stimulate curiosity about the patient's life, the discussion is well grounded in reality. A more serious objection, as mentioned above, is that Balint group work, like any form of supervision, is a slow process that needs commitment. In the case of GP trainees the regular inclusion of a group may be seen as eating up valuable time in a crowded curriculum. Our experience is that the trainees, while often doubtful of the group's value to begin with, end up regarding it as the most helpful part of their weekly teaching.

How long do people need a Balint group for?

As we have described, Balint's original groups met weekly for several years and were a very intensive experience. They were '*Research* cum training' (our italics) groups. Balint was at first very much against the idea of a more 'dilute' experience but later, as mentioned previously, he agreed to run a group for medical students. Even this, so far as Balint was concerned, was a research project.

Nowadays we do not feel there is any hard and fast rule as to how long people might want to be in a group for. Some people find the group experience so useful, they continue indefinitely. Others might have a limited Balint group experience such as attending a Balint Society weekend or taking part in a group as a GP trainee and they find this is sufficient to help their practice become more patient-centred.

So far as the groups themselves are concerned, their duration is very variable. We have already mentioned the Canadian group that is still going strong after over twenty-five years. At the other extreme, groups may come and go quite quickly, sometimes ending because of a fall off in membership. Groups for GP trainees will normally run continuously on the half-day release course with the trainees attending when they can (often difficult when in hospital posts) through their three years of GP training.

How are Balint group leaders trained and accredited?

Balint leaders in the UK should first of all have spent a substantial amount of time as a Balint group member. Ideally they should learn from working as an associate with an experienced leader for a suitable period, perhaps a year. The research tradition and ethos of Balint groups means that invariably the leaders will discuss the process of the groups and the leader interventions, thus helping the associate leader to acquire relevant skills.

It is not always easy for a potential leader to find an experienced leader to work with for a long period of time. An alternative form of training is attendance at an appropriate number of leader training weekend workshops, perhaps six, where potential leaders are able to co-lead with an experienced leader and discuss the process.

The UK Balint Society now has a system of accreditation in place (Council of the Balint Society 2009). In order to obtain accreditation leaders need to show that they have been through the sort of training described above, they must provide a reference from an accredited Balint group leader with whom they have co-led a group and they may be called for interview in order to demonstrate that they meet the criteria.

New group leaders need to arrange ongoing supervision for a suggested minimum period of two years. Obviously such supervision is also useful for more experienced leaders. Methods of supervision might include attendance at the Balint Society's group leaders' workshop (held three times a year in London) and presenting their group for discussion, attending residential weekend workshops for leader training or by correspondence with a supervisor.

How easy is it to join a Balint group?

There are a few ongoing Balint groups in the UK. Anyone wishing to join a group should check out the Balint Society website, www.balint.co.uk. This will provide the necessary contact details. If a nearby group is not available, the Society organizes a number of weekends of Balint groups in various parts of the country. Many people find that attending one or two weekends a year gives them a good, refreshing experience and avoids the need for a regular commitment back home.

Most Balint groups are now open to all and it is not necessary to go through an interview process before joining. Very occasionally some participants do not fit well into a group, perhaps because they have too rigid an approach. If they do not realize this themselves, the leader(s) may have to consider asking them to leave the group. However, this would be unusual as groups are able to tolerate and accept a range of different personalities.

In conclusion

We suggest that the Balint group was probably the first form of supervision for GPs that looked at the unique nature of their work. It is just as valuable a method now as it was when it started. Unfortunately the ethos of these groups is seen as running counter to the current 'evidence-based' culture, thus limiting their popularity, at least in the UK.

References

Balint, E. and Norell, J. (1973) *Six Minutes for the Patient*. London: Tavistock Publications.

Balint, M. (1957) *The Doctor, His Patient and the Illness*. London: Pitman.

Balint, M., Ball, D. and Hare, M. (1969) Training medical students in patient-centred medicine, *Comprehensive Psychiatry*, 10: 249–58.

Bryant, D. (2007) A Balint Group is not just for doctors, in *Medicine, Evidence and Emotions 50 years on. Proceedings of the 15th International Balint Congress*. Lisbon: Cor Expressa.

Campkin, M. (1986) Is there a place for Balint in vocational training?, *Journal of the Association of Course Organisers*, 1: 100–4.

Council of the Balint Society (1994) What is a Balint Group?, *Journal of the Balint Society*, 22: 36–7.

Council of the Balint Society (2009) The Balint Society guidelines for accreditation of Balint Group leaders, *British Journal of the Balint Society*, 37: 5.

Hawkins, P. and Shohet, R. (2000) *Supervision in the Helping Professions*, 2nd edn. Maidenhead: Open University Press.

Kjeldmand, D. and Holmström, I. (2008) Balint Groups as a method of increasing job satisfaction and reducing professional burnout among GPs, *Annals of Family Medicine*, 6: 138–45.

Pinder, R., McKee, A., Sackin, P. *et al.* (2006) *Talking About My Patient: The Balint Approach in GP Education*. Occasional Paper 87. London: Royal College of General Practitioners.

Salamon, M. (2009) The Ottawa Balint Group qualitative research project: a radical method of continuing education – exploring reflection, in International Balint Federation (ed.) *Proceedings of the 16th International Balint Congress*. Miercurea Ciuc, Romania: Alutus.

Salinsky, J. and Sackin, P. (2000) *What Are You Feeling, Doctor?* Oxford: Radcliffe.

Shoenberg, P. and Suckling, H. (2004) A Balint Group for medical students at Royal Free and University College School of Medicine, *Journal of the Balint Society*, 32: 20–3.

4 Narrative-based supervision

Helen Halpern and Sue Morrison

Editors' introduction

This is the first of three chapters written by trainers from the London Deanery who have extensive experience in the supervision of doctors. The skills they outline in this chapter on narrative-based supervision are founded on good listening and effective questioning, both of which are relevant to areas beyond supervision such as patient care. These skills can be developed relatively quickly and easily and as such this chapter offers a practical tool that those new to clinical supervision could 'try out' and illustrates a method that could be included as part of every doctor's routine of professional life. Through helping supervisees to develop new stories, they are advocating a form of reframing which we think is both a very useful life skill and a valuable professional tool. The philosophy behind their methodology, we believe, has much in common with the philosophy of the Balint group in its wish to let supervisees discover as much as possible for themselves. So although they might look like very different approaches, we can see in their respect for the supervisee's autonomy a similarity with the previous chapter.

Overview of chapter

In this chapter we give an outline of one of the theoretical and practical approaches to supervision. It provides a framework based on asking questions that develop the accounts of supervisees in order to help them move on from a problem or dilemma where they are feeling stuck. This method of supervision is useful for doctors as it can be used in brief encounters on the job as well as in more formal settings.

Introduction

This chapter will cover the background and theory of a model of narrative-based supervision that is taught by the London Deanery (the organization that is responsible for postgraduate medical and dental training in the London area which is being extended to other regions and countries). Narrative-based supervision provides a form of postgraduate education and training that is applicable to the whole medical profession and clinical team. It offers a model of supervision that is not just about imparting knowledge and skills but also helps to develop autonomy and reflective practice.

By the end of 2011 we had put on thirty, three-day courses in Supervision Skills for Clinical Teachers, alongside several hundred one-day courses at the London Deanery, as well as for trainers' groups, appraisers' groups and in secondary care Trusts. In addition, for the last three years we have run year-long courses to extend the skills of clinicians who are particularly interested in teaching and facilitating others in using narrative-based supervision within medical settings. These courses have introduced doctors to the ideas which have been called Conversations Inviting Change (Launer 2002). There is now a growing body of clinicians who meet and practise these skills in locally based groups and we continue to develop and write about the theoretical background to the model (Launer and Halpern 2006; Halpern 2009; Launer 2009a).

What is supervision?

There are many definitions of supervision. Our preferred version is that of supervision as a focused conversation about work that is aimed at developing professional practice and improving patient care. Supervision for doctors offers an opportunity to step back from the particular dilemma or situation and get a fresh perspective in order to work more effectively and safely. Supervision is an externalized version of reflective practice (Launer 2003).

Supervision for doctors fulfils a number of functions: normative, formative and restorative (Proctor 2001). The normative aspect relates to the managerial, benchmarking function of supervision, enabling supervisees to have a sense of how their work fits into the range of other doctors' work. The formative aspect of supervision is about the opportunity afforded for personal and professional development and education. The restorative aspect is that of supervision as a professional oasis, offering a breathing space for support and reflection. Although some doctors are naturally reflective, others are shy of this term. However, the ability to demonstrate reflective practice is increasingly required in trainees' learning portfolios: 'Reflection is the bridge between theory and practice; it is how experience is understood and converted into knowledge' (West-Burnham 2004).

Others have defined the function of supervision as promoting professional development through the functions of education, support and administration (Kilminster and Jolly 2000).

Postgraduate supervision for doctors

For many years all doctors in training have had a supervisor to oversee their work. Some would say the training of doctors was very much like an apprenticeship, but as well as this, some individual supervisors in primary and secondary care have developed a more reflective, narrative approach. From our background as GPs we have experience of this kind of high-quality supervision within GP training. This has spread more widely since 2000 and the standards for supervision in secondary care have also developed beyond the process of simply overseeing the trainee's practice. In training settings there is now a requirement for formal clinical and educational supervision of trainees (Gold Guide 2010). As well as the need to monitor competencies, supervision is becoming understood as a process of getting help from colleagues about a range of difficulties or issues related to work.

Although there has long been the recognition that in order to provide suitable supervision doctors need training, encouragement and support in the difficult task of both evaluating and valuing the work of their juniors (Hale 1992), the provision of such training for supervisors has been patchy. We should not assume that senior doctors, even those with many years of experience, will necessarily have the skills needed to provide appropriate supervision. The process can often be complicated as it may involve working with complex overlaps of clinical, ethical and personal areas as well as across the domains of development and performance. The General Medical Council (GMC 2003 and 2012) recognizes the importance of the development of such skills, and consultant trainers with a supervisory responsibility need training and ability in supervision (Swanwick 2009). In other words, supervision is a skill that can be taught and learnt and it should no longer be assumed that experience as a doctor is enough in itself to make a good teacher or supervisor.

There are a number of barriers to supervision including the perception that it is time-consuming, taking doctors away from the direct provision of a clinical service to patients. There may also be a feeling that supervision is only required for those whose skills are not yet adequate. However, our experience is that the need of senior doctors to discuss issues arising in everyday practice may be just as great as those of trainees. Continuing supervision after completion of training may help personal development, improve morale, aid the ability to support colleagues and promote the retention of staff.

As doctors become used to having higher quality supervision throughout their training there is an increasing likelihood that supervision will become embedded in professional development culture.

Different models of supervision for doctors

There are a number of models of supervision that can be used and several of these are covered in other chapters in this book.

The narrative-based model was developed by Launer and colleagues and has been described as 'conversations inviting change' (Launer 2002). In narrative-based supervision supervisees tell the story of the issue that they wish to bring, facilitated by the supervisor asking questions to help them make a shift in their thinking (Halpern

2009). Within a narrative-based model the supervisor takes a 'not knowing' approach (Anderson and Goolishian 1992: 25–39), aiming to turn his or her own hypotheses and assumptions into questions rather than offering interpretations. Although emotional issues may be discussed, the direct focus is not on the feelings of the supervisee and there is no supposition of getting to the bottom of things or to any particular core. With certain exceptions (legal, ethical or clinical governance concerns) the process is driven by the supervisee's agenda which may include his or her feelings along with a need to address a broader range of factors including the technical supervision of procedures. In contrast to some approaches (Cole 2002) this is not purely solution-focused but aims to enable the supervisee to develop a new narrative.

Background to narrative-based supervision

Narrative is about making sense of experience through dialogue with others. We believe that this model of narrative-based supervision is valuable within a medical context because such a conversation helps to create new understandings that can address the technical aspects of work *as well as* the ethical and human issues that arise in working with others and caring for patients. Narrative-based supervision has emerged from a base of narrative-based primary care. Over the last ten years or so, under the leadership of Dr John Launer, a group of clinicians has developed the application of narrative ideas for supervising doctors. The project began in the 1990s at the Tavistock Clinic in London, with a course for primary care clinicians, run by Dr Caroline Lindsey and Dr John Launer (Launer and Lindsey 1997). Participants on the course wanted to learn skills to discuss cases and work-based dilemmas. The course members were encouraged to think about the influences of family members, the clinical teams involved and the effects of financial and political contexts in the consultation. Some ideas from systemic family therapy (Palazzoli Selvini *et al.* 1980; Cecchin 1987; Tomm 1988) were blended with narrative approaches in medicine (e.g. Brody 1994; Frank 1998; Greenhalgh and Hurwitz 1998; Mattingly and Garro 2000; Charon and Montello 2002; Charon 2008; Kalitzkus and Matthiessen 2009). In particular we highlighted the use of curiosity, asking questions that could expand and enrich the clinician's story about the case. It became apparent that not only were narrative skills helpful in consultations with patients but that doctors could use the very same ideas in their conversations with colleagues to help develop new stories and better understanding of their experience.

There are three principles of this approach to narrative-based supervision (Launer 2009b):

1 All conversations are a form of shared storytelling.
2 Stories change through a process of dialogue.
3 People need to maintain ownership of their own stories.

Doctors are familiar with these principles in relation to consultations with patients where the patient's and doctor's stories shift through the conversation between them.

Similarly colleagues' stories can change through the supervision conversation to enable the supervisee to move from a stuck story (Andersen 1987) towards a new viewpoint. The supervision may end with an action plan created jointly by the supervisor and supervisee and ideally agreed and owned by the supervisee.

The basic methodology

The narrative model we have developed is based on a variety of questioning techniques derived from an influential group of family therapists known as the Milan team (Palazolli Selvini *et al.* 1980; Cecchin 1987; Tomm 1988). It is informed by three main principles:

1   Hypothesizing: supervisors will inevitably make assumptions and interpretations about what they hear. Turning these hypotheses into questions is a key skill in this approach. The supervisor needs to maintain an attitude of curiosity rather than certainty (Mason 1993) about what is necessarily right or best.

2   Circularity: by always framing questions as a response to what has already been said, the supervisor remains with the supervisee's narrative. Although this may guard against the supervisor probing into unwanted areas, it can occasionally be necessary to do this in some training situations, for example if there are concerns about patient safety and/or the competence of the clinician.

3   Neutrality: supervisors should use their curiosity about the supervisee's story to maintain a non-judgemental approach without betraying their opinions unless ethical or governance issues demand that they take a particular stance.

An example of narrative-based supervision

We give an annotated example of a piece of supervision that Danny, a consultant in Accident and Emergency medicine, had from a colleague, Lou, a consultant anaesthetist, in an educational supervisors' workshop. The conversation took about fifteen minutes. It is based on a real conversation but has been altered to preserve the anonymity of the people involved.

The dilemma in this piece of supervision is about personal interaction and emotion, which is the kind of topic that is frequently brought to supervision with colleagues. Note that only the supervisor ever asks questions. The questions are short and open. There is a sense of how each question follows on from the supervisee's previous response. The supervisor accepts the supervisee's story and does not offer any interpretations or advice, but allows the supervisee to come up with his own solution.

This example illustrates the type of conversational content and comments on the rationale behind the questions asked but obviously cannot convey other important contributions such as body language, intonation and tone of voice. There are always different options for what questions to ask and different routes to explore. There are no 'best' or 'right' questions. The supervisor will be guided by verbal and non-verbal feedback to tune in to those that seem to help develop the supervisee's thinking.

CASE EXAMPLE: LOU AND DANNY

Lou   *Could you tell me in a nutshell what would you like to talk about?* (The supervisor asks for a brief outline only. This can help the supervisee to focus on the nub of the issue.)

Danny   There's a new trainee who has recently joined the team. Some of the nurses have described him as having a bullying attitude.

Lou   *What more do I need to understand about the context and the players involved?* (The supervisor needs just enough detail to make sense of the problem. The supervisee will be the main judge of what the supervisor needs to know in order to help move things forward.)

Danny   It's a busy department. The experienced nurses resent the way that this person talks to them. They come and complain to me. They say that he's not respectful and has a patronizing attitude, especially to some of the younger nurses. He makes unreasonable requests for nurses to help him with procedures or to drop everything else to attend to his needs in a way that could be perceived as bullying or intimidating. I'm one of the consultants in the department, so I work with him at times, but I'm not his Educational or Clinical Supervisor. He's a really good doctor and I personally have no issues with him.

Lou   *Where would you like to be at the end of this conversation with me?* (This is an important question to ask early in the supervision to find out what the supervisee wants and to help crystallize the issue.)

Danny   To know where my loyalties lie and to have a plan for what to do.

Lou   *What makes you a key player in this?* (This helps the supervisee to reflect on his own part in the process.)

Danny   I'm one of the senior consultants in the department. I seem to get on well with him, even though other people don't have a good rapport with him. I also get on well with the people he's had problems with.

Lou: *Have you asked him why this is happening?* (This is quite a challenging question that helps to establish what the supervisee has already tried.)

Danny: I've been worried about doing that.

Lou: *If you were to tackle the issue, what kinds of questions would you ask him?* (The supervisor does not challenge him about his own response by asking 'what's stopped you?' but by asking a hypothetical question about what he might do, the supervisee can explore the possibility and this may allow him to decide whether or not that is the most appropriate course of action.)

Danny: I'd ask what I could do to be helpful.

Lou: *If this doctor's Educational Supervisor was here, what might they say about the situation?* (The supervisor now asks questions to get some other people's perspectives. This can help the supervisee to see the situation from different points of view.)

Danny	They'd say that it's like walking a tightrope between helping the trainee and helping the nurses, especially if anyone makes a formal complaint about bullying.
Lou:	*What about one of the senior nurses; what might they say?*
Danny	That everyone in the team needs to pull their weight and that this doctor's attitude is not sympathetic to the needs of other people in the team.
Lou	*What does 'pull their weight' mean?* (The supervisor tunes in to the supervisee's specific language and picks up a phrase that seems to be a cue for understanding the problem. The cue can be recognized by the supervisee's tone of voice – emotionally loading the words used, combined with his facial expression and the supervisor's curiosity about his own response to how he hears these particular words.)
Danny	Being aware of give and take; helping each other out, not just with the medical jobs; understanding that everyone's job is important.
Lou:	*How have they communicated that to him?* (The supervisor asks about the interaction between people.)
Danny:	There have been lots of abrupt comments, not always very diplomatic. I think it may be too late now to tackle the problem.
Lou:	*Is there a protocol within the department about who is responsible for tackling such problems?* (The supervisor appears to have a hypothesis that there is likely to be a protocol the supervisee could use but the naivety of this question may be face-saving for the supervisee who may not be sure. The supervisor might also have picked up on the cue 'I think it's too late now to tackle the problem' and this may have taken the supervision in a completely different direction. What other questions could the supervisor have asked at this point?)
Danny:	I think it's the Educational Supervisor but I need to check if there is a formal protocol.
Lou:	*How could you have a conversation about this in your department?* (This question implies that the supervisor thinks a departmental conversation might be helpful. The way the question is phrased, however, is non-authoritarian and invites thinking about the process of setting up such a conversation.)
Danny:	I should speak to the Educational Supervisor. You're right, I need to find out what I'd need to do to take things further, rather than just leave the situation to fester.
Lou:	*What kind of conversation would you want to have in the department?* (It is often helpful to invite supervisees to try what they might want to say. This can help them clarify the issues further by hearing themselves speaking the words.)
Danny:	How to use me to help build bridges between people to resolve things. I think I could help identify some of the potential stumbling blocks in getting people to work together and what measures to put in place. Even whether I am actually the right person to do the negotiating; perhaps it should be somebody else.

> Lou: *If the trainee had been listening in to our conversation so far what might he say?* (This is another alternative perspective question that can help to move the supervisee towards action through completing the circle of views.)
>
> Danny: That he'd want to be involved in some mediation process before anyone made a formal complaint of bullying against him. He'd want to understand the nurses' position. I think he'd be surprised that we've spent so much time talking about him.
>
> Lou: *How is this conversation going for you?* (Encouraging the supervisee to summarize can help the supervisor to judge the effectiveness of the supervision. It can be asked more than once in a piece of supervision. It may allow the supervision to go in a more useful direction if the supervisee is not finding it helpful or it can round off the supervision. The supervisee may wish to come up with some action points at this stage.)
>
> Danny: It's been useful to talk more about the situation. It's made it clearer that my loyalties are both to the trainee and to the others in the team. I do like this guy despite his behaviour, but it's also helped me clarify that I can't just ignore how things are. I need to talk more to some of the others involved, especially to his Educational Supervisor and I need to discuss with other people what they think my role should be in sorting this out. Thank you.

Although we outline the process here, the theory is less important than an open and facilitative attitude of mind combined with genuine curiosity about whatever dilemma the supervisee brings.

The structure of narrative-based supervision

- The supervisor has a conversation with the supervisee about an issue chosen by the supervisee.
- The supervisor uses a modified form of Socratic technique (mainly asking questions) based on material brought into the conversation by the supervisee.
- Ideally this generates a circular pattern of asking questions based on the supervisee's previous responses (see Figure 4.1).
- The supervisor pays close attention to the language used by the supervisee and uses the same words as far as possible in framing the next question. In addition the supervisor will enquire about the meaning of particular words and cues within the supervisee's narrative. This is similar to the concept of 'clean language' and the use of metaphor (Tomkins and Lawley 1997; Sullivan and Rees 2008).
- The supervisor will be curious about body language as well as verbal feedback as this will help to guide him or her in getting an appropriate balance between affirmation and challenge for the supervisee.

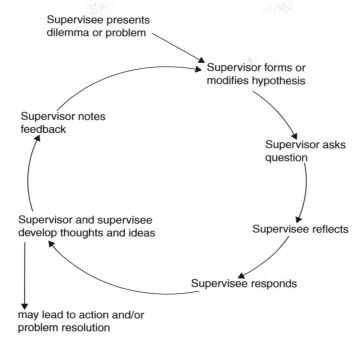

Figure 4.1 The circular process of supervision
Source: Halpern and McKimm 2010: 58)

- In this model, giving advice is kept to a minimum although it may be offered towards the end of a piece of supervision. Of course there are times when it may be necessary to give advice; some supervisees may need particular technical advice from a colleague who has more expert knowledge and there may be situations where the supervisor needs to give advice for legal, ethical or clinical governance reasons.

Below are some specific concepts which are useful for the supervisor to hold in mind during the supervision. Launer (2006: 19) has described these in a framework called The Seven Cs.

The Seven Cs

You may want to look back at the earlier supervision example and see how you think some of the Seven Cs fit with this.

- **Conversation:** an effective dialogue with others can create new ideas and help to promote a shift in thinking for a supervisee who is feeling stuck.

- **Curiosity:** curiosity is different from nosiness. It is important for supervisors to be non-judgemental and not to make assumptions. Instead, they will use their own experience and assumptions to form hypotheses which they check out by asking questions. The supervisor needs to be sensitive to cues from the supervisee in relation to enquiring about areas which he or she may feel are too personal.
- **Context:** this is often a fruitful area for curiosity. The supervision may cover many areas of context, especially those that affect the way that power is expressed and that may be affected by differences between people, e.g. gender, age, culture, sexuality, etc.
- **Complexity:** it is helpful to think that the connections between people and events are not linear but may be multilayered or form circular patterns. Seemingly simple issues brought to supervision can turn out to be quite complex and vice versa.
- **Creativity:** supervision can provide a forum for the development of new ideas through the exploration of multiple perspectives. This can create new views of the original issue brought to supervision and may be a more helpful way for the supervisee to move forward or manage that issue.
- **Caution:** the supervisor needs to balance an appropriate amount of challenge with support and affirmation of the supervisee.
- **Care:** it is important to ensure that the supervision process is carried out with mutual respect and sensitivity. Supervisors need to be aware of appropriate boundaries; their own as well as those of the supervisee.

The following case example is a reminder of the importance of balancing Caution and Challenge as well as Care in the Seven Cs; supervisors need to be aware of feedback and match what they offer to the particular supervisee and to the context. It can be a particular risk for supervisors with some psychotherapeutic training who may cross a boundary into offering therapy when it is not appropriate.

CASE EXAMPLE: KEITH AND KAREN

Keith, a radiologist, had supervision from Karen, a psychiatrist, in an educational supervisors' peer group facilitated by HH. Keith was aware that he had not yet given any feedback to a trainee who was not performing adequately and wanted help to think about why he found it hard to tackle the topic and how to do this effectively. Karen enquired about what factors might be stopping him from bringing up the problem with the trainee. Keith said that one of the difficulties was that the trainee seemed to be trying hard and was very pleasant. Karen then asked about gender issues and whether Keith was concerned about what the trainee might think about him. He thought that this was relevant as he wanted to be kind to his trainees and for them to like him. At this point Karen wanted 'to go for the jugular' (as she later described it) with her own idea that the supervisee's reluctance was related to the kind of parent he wanted to be to his trainee. This was Karen's interpretation and she gave it in an unsolicited way. Instead of following the model of turning this idea into a question, she started to explain her idea to Keith who gave very clear non-verbal feedback of extreme discomfort. We stopped here to ask how Keith was finding the supervision. He said that he had found it very helpful until then but that Karen's interpretation had felt inappropriate in this setting. The supervision then continued and followed Keith's request to rehearse some possible conversations he could have with the trainee.

A particular feature of the narrative-based model is that it is very supervisee-centred. Generally the supervisee determines what is brought for supervision. Frequently the outcome cannot be predicted in advance as in this narrative model this is created jointly in the conversation between supervisor and supervisee. At times the supervisor will need to intervene and take a more didactic approach if there are concerns about performance or training. The interplay between these ways of working is illustrated in Figure 4.2. If a supervisor finds that he or she needs to move from a developmental approach to focus more on performance it is important to flag this up to the supervisee.

CASE EXAMPLE: NATHAN

Nathan, a GP trainee, visited a patient at home before going to his GP study afternoon at the local postgraduate medical centre. At the end of the afternoon Nathan accidentally left his unlocked medical bag containing a printout of a patient's notes in the room. The postgraduate centre manager had found the bag and had telephoned the surgery to say that it was safe. The trainer, as supervisor, was able to use a developmental style with Nathan to review the care of the patient up to the point where Nathan did not seem to recognize the potential seriousness of leaving behind an unsecured bag containing confidential information. The trainer then had to explain that although Nathan had managed the patient's clinical care very well, they now needed to think about performance issues together. This allowed the trainer to continue to use a narrative, questioning style to get him to think further about his performance. For example: What if the postgraduate centre manager had read the patient's notes? What did Nathan know about the GMC position on breaches of confidentiality? Did Nathan have an ethical duty to let the patient know what has happened? What steps was he going to take to ensure that a similar situation was unlikely to be repeated? The conclusion of the supervision will depend on Nathan's responses to this last group of questions. If he realizes that he has made a serious error and is contrite, all the trainer need do is to acknowledge that he agrees. If, however, his answers continue to demonstrate a lack of insight the trainer will then need to make a clear statement. He will need to explain that on this occasion Nathan has not maintained an acceptable standard in relation to the duties of a doctor, to say how he should have performed and point out that there are potentially serious consequences.

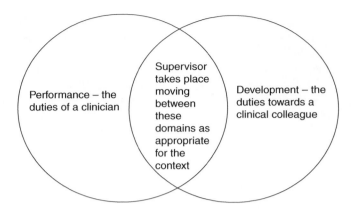

Figure 4.2 Diagram of performance and development

- **Super VISION** = performance – checking that patient care is carried out to the required professional standard and level of competence.
- **SUPER vision** = development – offering support and the opportunity for creativity and thinking outside the box.

What's the evidence?

One of the difficulties in providing evidence for the effectiveness of supervision is in deciding on what supervision processes should be evaluated and what outcomes to measure. It is also difficult to extrapolate information about the effects of supervision on patient care from the existing studies that have been carried out (Kilminster and Jolly 2000). The study of paediatric specialist registrars in North West London (Lloyd and Becker 2007) on their views of educational supervision showed that they found feedback on performance, careers advice, objective setting and pastoral support of value but overall did not find the type of supervision that they received to be particularly helpful. This may reflect the expectations of the trainees and the skills of the supervisors and could indicate a need for further training in supervision skills for both groups. This seems to support the need for widespread training in supervision skills and for it to become embedded as part of ongoing professional work.

Mendel and colleagues (2009) discuss the evidence supporting the value of supervision for doctors. Supervision can be useful both in learning networks (see Chapter 6) and with individuals.

Griffin *et al.* (2010) report that newly qualified GPs want the support of peers and/or mentors and some form of continuity or extended assistance that deals with the issues of a changing role. Kennedy *et al.* (2007) recognize that

> . . . the effects of increased supervision on patient care and trainee education are not known, primarily because the current multifaceted and poorly operationalized concept of clinical supervision limits the potential for evaluation.

This fits with our experience and concerns and in the chapter on appraisal (Chapter 9) we consider how the use of supervision can have a positive effect on patient care.

We have descriptive evidence of how colleagues across the range of medical specialties have applied their learning in this supervisory method in their clinical work. For example:

Hospital consultant:	*I have been trying to observe and practise the use of different questioning styles in conversations with trainees, colleagues and patients and also to notice when I am being supervised and my ideas are challenged.*
GP principal:	*I have used the skills when management dilemmas are brought to me. I am now less likely to jump in and do and more likely to facilitate thinking around the issue.*

Summary

We have given a brief outline of narrative-based supervision in medical settings. Some applications of the central theme of conversations inviting change are developed and explored further in Chapters 6 and 9. We have included some detailed case studies to give a flavour of the technique. However, we would encourage readers to try using some of the approaches in supervision sessions to get a fuller appreciation of this way of working.

References

Andersen, T. (1987) The general practitioner and consulting psychiatrist as a team with 'stuck' families, *Family Systems Medicine*, 5(4): 468–81.

Anderson, H. and Goolishian, H. (1992) The client is the expert: a not-knowing approach to therapy, in S. McNamee (ed.) *Therapy as Social Construction*. London: Sage Publications.

Brody, H. (1994) 'My story is broken: can you help me fix it?' Medical ethics and the joint construction of narrative, *Literature and Medicine*, 1: 79–92.

Cecchin, G. (1987) Hypothesizing, circularity and neutrality revisited: an invitation to curiosity, *Family Process*, 26(4): 405–13.

Charon, R. (2008) Narrative evidence based medicine, *Lancet*, 371: 296–7.

Charon, R. and Montello, M. (2002) *Stories Matter: The Role of Narrative in Medical Ethics*. London and New York: Routledge.

Cole, M. (2002) Appraising your colleagues, *BMJ Careers*, 18 May: 156–7.

Frank, A. (1998) Just listening: narrative and deep illness, *Families, Systems and Health*, 16(3): 197–212.

General Medical Council (2003) *Tomorrow's Doctors*. London: General Medical Council.

General Medical Council (2012) *Leadership and Management for All Doctors: Supervision*. Subsections 60, 61 and 62. Available at: http://www.gmc-uk.org/guidance/ethical_guidance/11826.asp.

Gold Guide (2010) *A Reference Guide for Postgraduate Specialty Training in the UK*, 4th edn. Available at: http://www.mmc.nhs.uk/pdf/Gold%20Guide%202010%20Fourth%20Edition%20v08.pdf.

Greenhalgh, T. and Hurwitz, B. (1998) *Narrative Based Medicine: Dialogue and Discourse in Clinical Practice*. London: BMJ Books.

Griffin, A., Abouharb, T., Etherington, C. and Bandura, I. (2010) Transition to independent practice: a national enquiry into the educational support for newly qualified GPs, *Education for Primary Care*, 21(5): 299–307.

Hale, R. (1992) The cobbler's children: how the medical profession looks after its own, *British Journal of Hospital Medicine*, 47(6): 405–7.

Halpern, H. (2009) Supervision and the Johari Window: a framework for asking questions, *Education for Primary Care*, 20(1): 10–14.

Halpern, H. and McKimm, J. (2010) Supervision, in J. McKimm and T. Swanwick (eds) *Clinical Teaching Made Easy: A Practical Guide to Teaching and Learning in Clinical Settings*. Herne Hill: Quay Books.

Kalitzkus, V. and Matthiessen, P. (2009) Narrative-based medicine: potential, pitfalls and practice, *The Permanente Journal*, 13(1): 80–6.

Kennedy, T., Lingard, L., Baker, R., Kitchen, L. and Regehr, G. (2007) Clinical oversight: conceptualizing the relationship between supervision and safety, *Society of General Internal Medicine*, 22: 1080–5.

Kilminster, S. and Jolly, B. (2000) Effective supervision in clinical practice settings: a literature review, *Medical Education*, 34(10): 827–40.

Launer, J. (2002) *Narrative Based Primary Care*. Oxford: Radcliffe.

Launer, J. (2003) Practice, supervision, consultancy and appraisal: a continuum of learning, *British Journal of General Practice*, 53(493): 662–5.

Launer, J. (2006) *Supervision, Mentoring and Coaching: One-to-one Learning Encounters in Medical Education*. Edinburgh: Association for the Study of Medical Education.

Launer, J. (2009a) Super vision, *Postgraduate Medical Journal*, DOI: 10.1136/pgmj.2009.082834.

Launer, J. (2009b) In the service of care and healing: an educator's viewpoint, in *Humanism and the Healing Arts: Transforming the Illness Experience – Patient and Practitioner Viewpoints*. Akron, OH: Institute for Professionalism Inquiry.

Launer, J. and Halpern, H. (2006) Reflective practice and clinical supervision: an approach to promoting clinical supervision among general practitioners, *Work Based Learning in Primary Care*, 4: 69–72.

Launer, J. and Lindsey, C. (1997) Training for systemic general practice: a new approach from the Tavistock Clinic, *British Journal of General Practice*, 47: 453–6.

Lloyd, B. and Becker, D. (2007) Paediatric specialist registrars' views of educational supervision and how it can be improved: a questionnaire study, *Journal of the Royal Society of Medicine*, 100(8): 375.

Mason, B. (1993) Towards positions of safe uncertainty, *Human Systems: The Journal of Systemic Consultation and Management*, 4: 189–200.

Mattingly, C. and Garro, L. (2000) *Narrative and the Cultural Construction of Illness and Healing*. Berkeley, Los Angeles, CA and London: University of California Press.

Mendel, D. *et al.* (2009) http://www.faculty.londondeanery.ac.uk/professional-development-framework-for-supervisors/pilot-evaluation-report.

Palazzoli Selvini, M., Boscolo, L., Cecchin, G. and Prata, G. (1980) Hypothesizing-circularity-neutrality: three guidelines for the conductor of the session, *Family Process*, 19(1): 3–12.

Proctor, B. (2001) Training for the supervision alliance attitude, skills and intention, in J. Cutliffe, T. Butterworth and B. Proctor (eds) *Fundamental Themes in Clinical Supervision*. London and New York: Routledge.

Sullivan, W. and Rees, J. (2008) *Clean Language: Revealing Metaphors and Opening Minds*. Carmarthen: Crown House Publishing.

Swanwick, T. (2009) Teaching the teachers: no longer an optional extra, *British Journal of Hospital Medicine*, 70(3): 126–7.

Tomkins, P. and Lawley, J. (1997) http://www.cleanlanguage.co.uk/articles/articles/109/1/Less-Is-More-The-Art-of-Clean-Language/Page1.html.

Tomm, K. (1988) Interventive interviewing: part III. Intending to ask lineal, circular, strategic, or reflexive questions?, *Family Process*, 27(1): 1–15.

West-Burnham, J. (2004) Building leadership capacity: helping leaders learn. Learning resource, pp. 1–6. National College for School Leadership, Nottingham.

5 Incidental supervision

Guy Undrill

Il faut cultiver notre jardin.

(Voltaire, *Candide*)

Editors' introduction

This is the first of two chapters where we look at alternatives to more formal sessions with a designated supervisor, the next one being about peer groups. In fact many doctors have said they do not need formal supervision as they get it in this informal way. We think that for this kind of supervision to be effective and not collusive considerable skills and experience are needed, perhaps even more than in more formal settings, to prevent it seeming as though the supervisee is just being told what to do. When provided in a hierarchical setting supervision can seem to focus more on, or be confounded by, educational or managerial priorities. It is also often one of the first things to be sacrificed because of pressure of time. Having said that, in emphasizing an egalitarian approach built on an inherent belief in supervisee competency, the writer highlights many of the issues that can come up and suggests ways of dealing with them. The chapter invites readers to glimpse what can be achieved by inspirational workplace supervision.

Overview of chapter

In this chapter, I look at how a supervisory stance can be helpful in day-to-day practice. When alert to the opportunities, there are frequent chances for brief supervisory interventions in everyday clinical work. The skills needed to use these opportunities safely, constructively and succinctly without interfering with the flow of clinical work differ in a few minor but important ways from the skills used in formal, scheduled supervision. This chapter looks at those differences. Although some of the skills needed are relatively advanced, the approach is particularly useful where there is minimal institutional support for formal supervision.

Why incidental supervision?

Incidental supervision is a modified form of supervision that is flexible, opportunistic and folded into practice. Doctors are familiar with the idea of informal bedside learning. Incidental supervision uses the same tactic to succinctly address puzzling or challenging aspects of a presentation on ward rounds, in clinics or home visits. It should be a brief intervention that has an immediate impact without breaking the flow of the primary clinical task. It is no substitute for properly contracted, regular supervision. However, in situations where supervision isn't institutionally supported, many of the needs that clinical supervision meets remain. Incidental supervision has two simple aims: to build the capacity to give and receive supervision in teams, and to regularly use brief interventions to keep teams focused on continuous improvement in clinical practice. It isn't a substitute for training in supervisory practice, and in some respects requires a greater sensitivity to power differentials than formal supervision, where issues of power should be explicitly addressed as part of contracting.

It is a sad fact that in the British National Health Service, there can be a widespread cultural hostility to supervision. Various factors drive this: supervision is often seen as a luxury, as a distraction from the main business of seeing patients in a time-pressured environment. Relationship-driven supervision often plays second fiddle to supervision as caseload management (particularly true of nurses) or supervision as educational supervision with endless electronic monitoring forms and 'workplace-based assessments' to grind through (particularly true of medical doctors). Where professional groups do aspire to embedding high quality clinical supervision into their practice they can be derided by other groups for taking an elitist, ivory-tower approach to work (particularly true of psychologists). Coupled with this, experiences of poor supervision are sometimes easier to come by than experiences of good supervision, and many clinicians will have experience of insensitively given feedback or crass interpretations of their own motivations, often given by people in positions of institutional power over them. This is invariably a highly aversive experience.

In place of contracting

In the wider world, a contract provides an agreement between two people that is of mutual benefit. A common feature of contracts is a balancing of power between the two parties so that the weaker party has some kind of guarantee that the stronger party won't misuse his or her position. This power rebalancing is a key feature of contracting in supervision, and the issues that are usually addressed around expectations and confidentiality are on one level there to protect both parties, but particularly the supervisee, from the consequences of asymmetries in power. For example, if a supervisee does not realize from a clear contracting process that there are limits to confidentiality and the supervisor feels that confidentiality needs to be broken (e.g. on an issue of professional competence), this could be experienced as a betrayal of confidence. Contracting has become an essential part of good standard supervisory practice: typically, when difficult issues arise in supervision, the contractual agreement is an essential part of resolving the issues, either by referring back to the original contract or by explicitly recontracting.

Providing supervision without a formal contract opens up some potential dangers, and these dangers are generally located in the area of asymmetries of power. In the absence of a contract to supervise, an incidental supervisor needs to be very mindful of power differentials and, as far as possible, to aim to minimize them. The spirit of the supervision should be egalitarian so that thinking about patients together becomes a collaborative enquiry between equals in the service of better clinical practice.

Approaching supervision as an egalitarian conversation can be difficult for people who have been trained and acculturated to hierarchical systems. In order to shift to a more egalitarian perspective, it is often helpful to think in terms that approach supervisees with a competence rather than deficit worldview:[1] see Table 5.1.

The deficit worldview is usually accompanied by a power differential as the person with the power is given the social authority to name the deficit and prescribe the remedy. A power imbalance coupled with a deficit worldview is usually at the root of poor quality supervision, whether formal or incidental. In formal supervision, issues of power are dealt with partly through contracting. In incidental supervision, this isn't an

Table 5.1 Deficit and competence approaches compared

Deficit worldview	Deficit worldview intervention	Competence worldview	Competence worldview intervention
The supervisee doesn't see the problem: there is denial or lack of insight.	Provide insight. Hold a mirror up to their faults.	The supervisee has a sense of professional curiosity about his or her practice.	Cultivate professional curiosity and seek the supervisee's insights.
The supervisee doesn't know: there is a knowledge deficit.	Provide facts.	Knowledge is within the supervisee.	Evoke the supervisee's knowledge.
The supervisee doesn't know how: there is a skills deficit.	Teach new skills.	The supervisee already has transferable skills which he or she can apply in his or her work.	Evoke the skills they use to identify them, reflect on them and generalize their scope.
The supervisee doesn't care.	Shame or frighten people into changing their practice.	The supervisee is highly motivated to develop professionally.	Enhance the supervisee's sense of self-efficacy.

option, and a careful adherence to a competence model is strongly recommended as a counterbalance to any institutional power the supervisor may have over the supervisee.

Using a competence model also builds a sense of safety in the supervisee to use supervision. Another way to build safety is to explicitly ask permission: asking permission is akin to making a contract in miniature. Anything that may come up in a contract can be part of asking permission: so a contract would normally deal with timings. In incidental supervision it might be appropriate just to ask permission to take some time out of a busy ward round to look at an issue: 'Would it be ok if we took five minutes to step back and look at this from a different perspective?' A contract would normally deal with boundaries and the practicalities of supervision. In incidental supervision we might make a request that is framed as an invitation. For example: 'Something seems to have made you angry about your encounter with Mr Smith. How would you feel about spending a few minutes looking at your feelings so that they don't get in the way of his treatment?' Needless to say, the question should be framed in a way that communicates it is genuine: the supervisee should feel comfortable to reply, 'Can we park that to a day when we're a bit quieter?' or, 'It's ok, I'll be fine after I've been for a run tonight.'

Because there is no formal contract, some of the things that one might contract for are absent, and these areas need a little more care. Particular caution needs to be exercised around interpreting what might be seen as the supervisee's unconscious behaviour (corresponding to supervision in Hawkins and Shohet's (2006) mode 5 and 6 supervision). Interpretation can be highly intrusive when not specifically contracted for: claiming that words mean something other than they were intended to mean risks 'hermeneutic violence', where the supervisor claims the position of the arbiter of meaning of the supervisee's words from a position of power. This can be followed by a withdrawal or closing down by the supervisee.

The competence worldview is of course not limited to incidental supervision, and applies very well in both formal supervision and in interactions with patients, where clinical interventions are often poorly contracted leaving patients feeling 'done to'.

Techniques and interventions

1 Be the supervisee

One of the strongest interventions for building supervisory capacity in teams is to be prepared to have incidental supervision from your own team. Senior doctors in positions of authority within teams are powerfully positioned to model how to deal with their own stuckness, ignorance or puzzlement. The benefits of asking for incidental supervision in this way are multiple: showing your own vulnerability straight away begins to level the power differential that can be difficult for supervision in the absence of a clear contract. It communicates that being puzzled is part of the job, and legitimizes this in the team's culture, which has some real benefits in terms of patient safety.

'Going first' as a supervisee allows you to address some of the aspects of supervision that might be more threatening to people unused to supervision, such as examining negative reactions to patients. For example, one could go to one's team and ask, 'I've really been rattled by my last patient in a way that doesn't usually happen to me. Can we quickly talk through what this might be about?': describe the patient (mode 1);

describe what you did (mode 2); think about the transference (mode 3) and describe your own reaction to the patient (mode 4) (modes 1 to 4 of the Hawkins and Shohet seven-eyed process model; Hawkins and Shohet 2006: 80–102).

'Being the supervisee' and asking for feedback also allows you to model how to respond to feedback. In particular, try not to be reactive or defensive and to listen to the feedback all the way through before responding. Treat what is said to you as an opinion and not the truth.

The last reason for 'being the supervisee' is not the least. Your team will invariably make a real effort to help you out and they will succeed more often than not.

2 Listen

Listening is a two-stage skill for the incidental supervisor. First, listen for opportunities for supervision. This often involves what psychotherapists (following Reik 1948) call 'listening with the third ear' – a kind of attention to what is implied or unsaid. In a team meeting, has the temperature of the room suddenly seemed to change? In a ward round that was going so well, do you suddenly feel bogged down? These might be opportunities for supervision.

Supervisor:	*We've got to the end of the round and left no time to see Mrs Jones again.*
Supervisee:	*We do need to see her . . .*
Supervisor:	*A 'but' is hovering in the air.*
Supervisee:	*She's just . . . draining. I don't think I've got the energy left this morning. And I'm starving hungry.*
Supervisor:	*Neither of us wants to see her. We conspire to minimize her opportunity to suck the lifeblood from us by squeezing her out of our timetable. You know, I sometimes think people are like that because they've learned it's the only way they can get what they need.*
Supervisee:	*There's a link there. Do you remember she said how her mother had to work three jobs to look after her and her five sisters? How her mother provided for them all but was just dog tired all the time and never actually played with them?*
Supervisor:	*You think we might be recreating her family of origin in the ward rounds. That's an interesting thought: it's almost like we're retraumatising her. OK, so what do you think we should do differently?*

The second stage is to listen to the actual content as it is brought to you: it is something of a cliché that listening is an active process. In listening, give the supervisee back little paraphrases and summaries of what they say. The skill in doing this is to highlight what seems important to help the supervisee sort unstructured impressions into a more coherent understanding of their patient.

3 Don't do it

Once you've got your ear tuned in to opportunities to supervise, let most of them go – after all, you haven't contracted to provide them any supervision at all. If a supervisory intervention has popped into your head, work through a check list: is this the right time and place? Is this the right issue? How safe does the supervisee feel with me?

Listen closely to your supervisees and they will teach you when to use this technique. They will invariably point out (with varying degrees of directness, from toe tapping to tears) when you have missed an opportunity to use it.

Although this intervention may seem a negative one – exercising restraint – using it can create the awareness and the space for other more appropriate 'holding' interventions. If this isn't the right time and place: when might be? Make a mental note to return to the issue. If this isn't the right issue: what is? Are there other aspects of the supervisee's practice that need attention first? If the supervisee doesn't feel safe with me: how can I build safety? All of these interventions require a longer-term view of the supervisee's development than just the issue at hand.

4 Ask permission

If you are going to make a supervisory intervention, ask permission. Asking permission is a skill in itself, and it should normally be framed in a tentative, provisional way to keep the supervisee safe. 'I've got an idea of a parallel process that might be going on here. Can I tell you about that?' or, 'I've got an idea here which may or may not help – is it OK if I share it with you?' or, 'I've seen something similar to this in the past with another clinician I used to work with – would you be interested to hear what he found helpful?' If what you have spotted seems critical, give the piece of information you need, but in such a way that the supervisee is given permission to disregard it: 'If this doesn't work for you, then feel free to ignore it, but I've sometimes found in this situation that...'.

In asking permission, aim to be transparent that what you are doing is a supervisory intervention. This doesn't have to be laboured, it can be simply a matter of marking out what one is doing as taking a moment to get some perspective on the hurly burly of everyday practice: 'In the past, I've found the busier I feel, the more I've benefited from taking a step back to reflect – can we take a couple of minutes to do that now?'

5 Privilege enquiry as your principal intervention

Approaching supervision with a competence rather than a deficit worldview means that good quality questions become your principal intervention as you try to evoke solutions, skills and knowledge from supervisees. As a rule of thumb, don't give information unless you've tried your best to elicit it first. Good, open questions allow supervisees to explore the sense of what they are doing, and should in some sense expand the scope of their understanding of the problem.

6 Move from particular to general to particular

The main purposes of incidental supervision are to help supervisees in the here and now and to build capacity for supervision. Help them to see how the particular issue they are wrestling with today might generalize to a principle they can apply again.

Supervisor: So, let me check through with you what happened here. You took a fairly immediate dislike to this man, and that disconcerted you slightly. What do you think was going on there?

Supervisee: I'm not sure what you mean...

Supervisor: Well, one of the things I've found makes this work easier is becoming aware of our own patterns and intuitions. Intuitions are often rather personal and you have to work out the patterns for yourself, because the way your intuitions work is going to be different to the way mine work. Didn't you have a similar reaction to someone a few weeks back? Is there a pattern?

Supervisee: There might be...I think both of them were hitting their partners...

Supervisor: So it might be that you're quite sensitive to this kind of violence and you're picking it up at a subconscious level before the patient's actually told you? There's some kind of alarm bell going off for you?

Supervisee: Maybe...do you know, now you mention it, I think I can remember another time that same thing happened. What's really strange is that with this patient it happened so instantly, like almost as soon as he'd walked in the door. He didn't even look like the sort of man who would harm a fly – but that was what he was so ashamed of, and what we got to forty minutes into the assessment.

Supervisor: That could be quite a useful thing to remember. If you catch yourself forming an instant dislike to a patient seemingly for no good reason, it might be a signal to you to pay attention to your feelings and to be aware there may be issues of domestic violence.

7 Focus on values

Moving away from a deficit model to a competence model (see Table 5.1) can be hard for people coming from a medical background for whom 'the patient is the one with the disease' (Shem 1978). When a supervisee is expressing frustration with a patient in deficit terms, a focus on values can help the supervisee see the patient's action as expressing a particular ethical stance, which can in turn open up other avenues to therapeutic opportunities. Often, this is best done in steps from behaviour to motivation to underlying values:

Supervisee: This man is an idiot. He knows that if he keeps drinking the amount he is drinking his liver is going to pack up and yet he just doesn't want to do anything about it. (The patient is viewed as lacking knowledge and motivation, with the implication that this is shameful.)

Supervisor: What do you think he gets out of his drinking? (Open question, refocuses from behaviour to motivation, assuming the patient has made a competent decision at some level.)

Supervisee: I did ask him that. All his friends go to the pub, and it gets him out of the house. He says that if he didn't do that, he'd argue with his wife.

Supervisor: A key part of his life is seeing his friends. It also seems important to him to look after his marriage – not to argue with his wife (paraphrasing what the supervisee has just said so that the supervisee hears it). What do you think this reflects in terms of his values? (Open question, explicitly asking about values.)

Supervisee: *He's a very social chap, his friends are important. I guess his family are impor-tant to him as well.* (A statement of the patient's values and strengths.)

Supervisor: *You've got a good idea of what's important to him in life.* (Validation of the supervisee's skills – an observation statement in the scheme below.) *Any kind of treatment we offer needs to respect and work with that.* (Explicit statement about the importance of values.) *What might you do next time you see him?* (Open question, shifting to action.)

Supervisee: *I don't think I really know enough about what's going on with his family. They seem both part of the problem and in some sense part of the solution. I need to explore that with him after the ward round.* (The supervisee comes up with an action plan autonomously.)

8 Affirm and validate

Validating supervisee behaviour well is harder than it looks. Vaughn Keller of the Health Services Research Center at the University of Miami (personal communication)[2] divides affirmation statements into *judgement*, *impact* and *observation* statements: see Table 5.2).

Particularly for the incidental supervisor, working towards an egalitarian relation-ship, judgement statements should be used more sparingly and impact and observation statements preferred. The following is a continuation from the case of Mrs Jones men-tioned on page 66.

Supervisee: *Well, one thing we could do differently is to see her at the beginning of the ward round. On a full stomach.*

Supervisor: *OK, and what will we do then?* (Open question.)

Supervisee: *Um . . . play with her?*

Supervisor: *OK, so you've seen a parallel process where she hasn't had her growth needs met in the past which we've unwittingly replicated in ward rounds and your impulse is to be playful, to give her the experience she didn't have as a child – a kind of corrective emotional experience if you like.* (Unpacks the supervisee's flip remark to find the truth in it and generalizes it to a psychotherapeutic principle.) *I like the way you're going with this* (impact statement), *let's run with the idea some more. What might it look like if we were more playful in our interactions with her?* (Open question incorporating a minor reframe of 'play with her' to 'more playful in our interactions'.)

9 Look after the process and the content will (almost) look after itself

This principle is sometimes also expressed as 'the wisdom is in the room'. When in a leadership position in a team, focus your interventions on process to allow all the knowledge, experience and insight of the team to be brought to bear on the issue at hand. As patients are being discussed, resist the temptation to offer 'the' answer but instead, aim to draw all members of the team into the discussion. A useful tip here is to ask the opinions of more junior members of the team first so that they feel less intimidated: they may still have information that is helpful to the group's

Table 5.2 Types of affirmation

	Description	Advantages	Disadvantages
Judgement	Supervisor makes a judgement of value from a position of authority (praise).	Useful with unconfident supervisees. Can be a helpful form of feedback in learning a new skill.	A power dynamic is introduced where the supervisor sets him/herself up as an expert in the supervisee's work. The supervisee doesn't have the opportunity to judge for him/herself whether something is good. At worst, judgement statements come across as patronizing. They can lead to resistance or irritation with the supervisor.
Impact	Supervisor describes the supervisee actions and then his or her own subjective positive response.	Impact statements are personal and can build rapport. Done well they can show to the supervisee that his or her actions have an effect on the supervisor, which can lead to a more equal relationship.	Because they are personal, they can shift focus unhelpfully on to the supervisor. They are easy to misjudge and can either go 'over the top' or not resonate with the supervisee.
Observation	Objective description of the supervisee's achievements as data.	The objectivity can balance out talk focused on deficits. The supervisee gets the credit for successes.	Can seem cold, clinical or removed.

decision-making process – for example, students may spend much more time with patients than more senior members of staff and may have more detailed knowledge of a patient's history. Where there is dissent in opinions on diagnosis or treatment, summarize both sides of the argument accurately and ask for comments. Paradoxically, the more one focuses on process/supervisory interventions and the less one relies on expert knowledge, the easier it is to be the senior person in the room. Even when a decision does fall to you, the quality of the debate that precedes the decision is far better if it is facilitated with a supervisory mindset, and this helps you to a better decision.

Structuring a piece of incidental supervision

In *Supervision in the Helping Professions*, Hawkins and Shohet (2006: 61–3) use the mnemonic CLEAR (Contract, Listen, Explore, Action, Review) to describe their model of supervision. In the absence of formal contracting, the following structure can be used in incidental supervision:

Listen: have you just heard an opportunity to make a supervisory intervention?

Evaluate: is this the right issue? Is this the right context? How secure is our relationship? (i.e. how safe does the supervisee feel with me?)

Timing: is now the right time?

Permission: ask for permission to make an observation, ask a question or make a suggestion.

Expand: use questions to expand the supervisee's understanding.

Action: ask the supervisee what he or she plans to do.

Review: arrange to review the decision.

Learning: what can be generalized from this specific situation?

For people who enjoy acronyms, this can be summarized as: 'Do I need to LET this supervision opportunity pass, or is there a PEARL I can elicit?'

Development

I am indebted to Helen Mentha (personal communication) for the idea that the relationship of incidental supervision to formal supervision parallels the relationship of incidental gardening to regular gardening. There is regular gardening – the planning, preparing, tilling and planting – but gardens thrive best when there is also incidental gardening, when there are a few minutes' dead heading of plants in the evening or when passing a pot one stops for a moment to check the moisture of the soil and gives it a little water if it needs it. Crucially, incidental gardening is based on a deep knowledge of the whole undertaking of gardening, even if at that moment one is only attending to one small part of one process in the garden. It has to be both meaningful in itself and part of the overall undertaking: like incidental supervision, one doesn't start a job that's too big to finish in the five minutes one has. Even if you know the whole garden needs a major overhaul (there are organizational problems or a culture hostile to supervision) a little nip and nurture here and there can be helpful and worthwhile.

Perhaps most importantly, the best incidental gardeners are the best gardeners: they have taken the time to study and learn from others but they have also 'learned to see things from the plant's point of view'. They notice things in their garden on a day-to-day basis and time their interventions with care, flexibility and precision – but they may also at times act decisively and quickly to stop a small problem becoming bigger. Incidental supervision similarly requires a good repertoire of skills and a strong supervisory awareness: it isn't an easy option or a substitute for formal supervision and certainly shouldn't be seen as a way of avoiding training or practice in formal supervision.

Notes

1. This helpful distinction is often made in Motivational Interviewing, e.g. Miller and Moyers (2006), Corbett (2009), though is very much part of the positive psychology

approach. For a brief introduction to positive psychology see Seligman and Csikszentmihalyi (2000) and other articles in this special edition of *American Psychologist*.
2. Keller says that the idea originated several years ago in conversations with Ed Deci and Rich Ryan: 'We were discussing the idea of pride in something someone else did. Ed sensitized me to what we say, and don't say, to our children.'

References

Corbett, G. (2009) What the research says...about the MI 'spirit' and the 'competence worldview', *MINT Bulletin*, 15: 1, 3–5.

Hawkins, P. and Shohet, R. (2006) *Supervision in the Helping Professions*. Maidenhead: Open University Press.

Miller, W. R. and Moyers, T. (2006) Eight stages in learning motivational interviewing, *Journal of Teaching in the Addictions*, 5(1): 3–17.

Reik, T. (1948) *Listening with the Third Ear: The Inner Experience of a Psychoanalyst*. New York: Grove Press.

Seligman, M. E. P. and Csikszentmihalyi, M. (2000) Positive psychology: an introduction, *American Psychologist*, 55(1): 5–18.

Shem, S. (1978) *The House of God*. New York: Richard Marek Publishers.

6 Peer supervision

Sue Morrison and Helen Halpern

Editors' introduction

We are often asked about the differences between formal and peer supervision. Being ourselves in peer group supervision we are strong advocates and recognize the many practical benefits it offers and that are described in this chapter. We recognize that for many doctors the informal meetings they have with colleagues and peers is often the nearest they get to ongoing support and for some the easiest way into more explicit supervision is to develop their opportunities for peer support and supervision. Being able to switch roles has the huge advantage of helping to loosen hierarchical ways of being (and thinking) but may not come naturally if they have not been encountered in training. It also draws out some of the difficulties of peer supervision that include a possible confusion of roles, 'blind spots' shared by peers and a possible avoidance of more challenging interventions. The authors draw out what is involved in establishing peer supervision and explore a number of different ways of working with peers, both one-to-one and in groups.

Overview of chapter

We both value the opportunity to give and receive peer supervision and think that it can enhance the quality of our work. We have offered a simple framework that can help doctors provide peer supervision through more structured use of conversations. We think this kind of supervision is underused because doctors don't notice the opportunities for it to take place. We have suggested several different formats for peer supervision to be used in different contexts.

Introduction

Peer supervision is a non-hierarchical professional conversation that takes place be-tween colleagues about their work. It is non-hierarchical in the sense that peers can take turns in being either supervisor or supervisee. Rather than comparing anecdotes or giving direct advice, we believe that through using a question-based, narrative ap-proach, peers can make a real difference in helping each other think about issues that arise at work. There are multiple opportunities for formal and informal peer supervi-sion during the working day, ranging from a few snatched minutes to more formal settings in protected time. We believe that all clinicians can benefit from taking part in supervision which contributes to lifelong learning and professional development. Peer supervision can be used to extend reflective professional practice as ideas develop in new ways when expressed to a colleague who may add further dimensions through the appropriate use of support and challenge.

In this chapter we will describe a model for peer supervision and explain how it can be used by doctors working in a variety of clinical settings.

Background

Peer supervision can take place either informally or formally. Informal supervision may occur over a cup of coffee or in the corridor (see Chapter 5). Formal opportunities for peer supervision may be within protected time in established clinical networks or in a group who come together for professional development within their professional roles as a learning team (Clutterbuck 2006). Some examples are:

- GP trainers;
- clinical tutors;
- new practitioners, e.g. Royal College of General Practitioners First GPs (an initiative to support GPs in their first five years of practice; Taylor *et al.* 2010);
- self-directed learners;
- sessional GPs;
- retired doctors;
- appraisers;
- local supervision groups;
- mentors;
- consultant peer groups;
- faculty groups;
- programme directors.

Some doctors are concerned that supervision is time-consuming, taking them away from the direct need to provide a clinical service to patients. There may also be a feeling that supervision is only required for those whose skills are not yet adequate. However, brief, informal and effective supervision can occur almost anywhere (see Chapter 5). Skills for peer supervision can be used throughout a professional career and applied in ways that can be adapted to fit the particular working context. This means that doctors can make more efficient use of their time by dealing effectively with workplace issues and dilemmas. The skills also foster self-sufficiency and autonomy. These are important skills to master from undergraduate level as '[Trainees] must be prepared for the initial change they will face, of graduating from being a student and supervised employee to an independent clinical leader and potential employer.' (De Kare-Silver 2010). If doctors become used to having peer supervision throughout their training it is likely to become a natural part of their everyday practice. Speciality trainees in general practice in the UK need to demonstrate reflective practice through their entries in the e-portfolio and the value of reflection is increasingly recognized in other specialities. This personal reflection can be extended through a supervisory conversation with a peer that externalizes some of the thinking process. However, supervision should not be restricted to trainees as the needs of senior doctors to discuss issues arising in everyday practice may be just as pressing. Launer (2003) refers to the potential risk to patient safety of not having an opportunity to have a conversation with a colleague about work.

Why develop supervision?

In a recent article about the increasing need to professionalize medical education, Shrewsbury and Mohanna (2010) suggest that supervision and professional conversations have an important role beyond training: 'Where this support continues into the postgraduate phase, it will involve us all in a collegial approach to mutual support and respect, nurturing excellence within the profession as well as managing errors effectively and constructively.'

Peer supervision groups can address a number of areas:

- managing a complex and changing working environment;
- improving communication with patients, families, teams and organizations;
- supporting colleagues;
- helping with career development;
- managing effective ways of working clinically through sharing ideas and practice.

Peer supervision of cases and workplace issues can make an important contribution to other aspects of clinical work because supervision improves transferable generic conversational skills (see Figure 6.1).

Good supervision skills

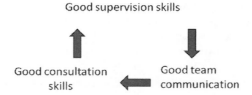

Good consultation skills   Good team communication

Figure 6.1 The virtuous circle of effective professional conversational skills in the clinical workplace

The provision of supervision throughout professional life also fits with the growing emphasis on developing leadership within healthcare. Peer supervision can help to develop and maintain leadership skills by supporting clinicians to take on challenges, to develop their own resources and by encouraging them to take appropriate responsibility for finding their own solutions to problems.

CASE EXAMPLE: MO

Mo, an obstetrician, asked for supervision in a multidisciplinary group of consultant colleagues. The hospital where he worked was being rebuilt and the ultrasound department was due to be located in a different building from the antenatal clinic. Mo felt that his arguments about the discomfort for patients with full bladders having to go some distance for their scans had been ignored. He described feeling angry and disempowered. This made him resentful towards the hospital management and reluctant to attend the forthcoming meeting with them and the architect. He described feeling stuck as he was concerned that his frustration might hold him back from taking any effective action. In supervision he was able to identify other colleagues who could be recruited to support his views. Mo was also able to rehearse how he would state his opinion at the meeting. He had feedback about the way he planned to present his views and also received considerable support from the other doctors present. Mo reported that this piece of supervision made him feel better prepared for the meeting.

The place of peer supervision

Peer supervision is not top-down, unlike many other areas in medicine. It is a mutual activity in which the supervisor can learn as much as the supervisee. Indeed, the doctor giving supervision to a colleague on one occasion may well subsequently receive supervision from that same colleague. (Some of these ideas were developed in the previous chapter.) This process can facilitate the professional growth of all those involved. This may happen directly, as supervisors, and indirectly as observers. Models of peer supervision within groups offer participants a number of ways to contribute to the process, including active observation. On some occasions they may have a role as witnesses to a process of change for the supervisee. Their diversity may be harnessed by using them as a reflecting team (Andersen 1987), offering observations and ideas to the supervisor and supervisee. The inclusion of observers in the process of supervision is also important from an educational perspective. For some doctors who may be wary of participating in experiential learning, perhaps related to their previous history of learning through humiliation, taking the observer-role can be a way of encouraging engagement and gaining confidence for more vulnerable or self-contained people.

CASE EXAMPLE: ADAM

Adam, a consultant paediatrician, sought advice from another consultant, Liz, about how to engage junior team members more in ward rounds. Adam was aware that he liked to teach using witty anecdotes about cases he had managed and that he had a reputation for being very knowledgeable. Liz suggested that Adam might get others involved more if he stopped being didactic and instead asked his colleagues questions. When he tried this the other team members were reticent to respond and the atmosphere in the ward rounds become quite hostile. This time Adam asked Liz for supervision about the issue and requested that instead of giving him advice, she should help Adam explore some different hypotheses and perspectives. She asked about different possible educational approaches, about his power and status in the team and the effects these factors might have. Adam recognized that the task was more complex than he had originally thought and that this realization was helpful in itself without necessarily having to change anything at this point. The conversation was also useful for Liz who realized that her approach of teaching by asking questions and rarely supplying answers could be perceived as equally unhelpful to learners.

This example also demonstrates a transitional stage, from an educational contract where the consultant knows best to a more egalitarian frame where both peers acknowledge that they have something to learn.

When clinicians from the same speciality supervise each other familiarity with the working context can be helpful as a shortcut but can also mean unhelpful assumptions may be made. Supervision from someone less familiar with the specific context can avoid this problem through his or her ability to ask 'naive' questions.

Some people quickly pick up skills in asking questions and tracking the supervisee's story; others struggle over a longer period to develop the technique. One of the most challenging aspects of this approach is not to rush in with advice and solutions. The process may be particularly difficult for clinicians working in highly technical specialities who have been trained to 'fix' problems. Peer supervision may provide a safe environment for learning and as a place where clinicians can offer each other feedback.

These peer supervision groups may be structured with pairs working one-to-one, or with one or more observers whose role is to provide a wider view on the supervision process (e.g. how the conversation is happening and what is and is not being talked about) as well as on the content of what is being discussed. This is considered in more detail later in the chapter.

In a peer supervision group part of the learning comes from the recognition of the influences of group interactions as well as incorporating individual learning processes (Falk, cited in Kilpatrick 1997). A group setting offers opportunities for clinicians to increase their ability to understand complexity and to develop their thinking in new ways, through accessing the multiple perspectives available through dialogue with others. This not only applies to patient care but can also help them manage the rapidly changing scene of working in the National Health Service through considering different ways of understanding the influences of politics, finance and power. Taking part in supervision with clinical colleagues within the work environment, particularly in an atmosphere of turbulence and change, can provide the chance for individuals and the organization to change together, co-creating new possibilities for the future (Obholzer 1994). Some advantages of peer supervision in groups are:

- it provides an opportunity for making links with other colleagues;
- it is a way to support the professional development of colleagues;
- it can be a safe environment for practising and cascading supervision skills;
- it models an effective and respectful way of discussing work-based dilemmas;
- learning can take place through observation of others;
- there is the potential for sharing a wide range of ideas and experience;
- it provides exposure to a variety of practices and conundrums;
- there is the chance to develop a cohort of clinicians for the future with transferable skills;
- it offers the possibility of cost saving by working with groups rather than individuals;
- it gives an opportunity for individuals to influence the organization within which they work;
- it can improve job satisfaction and morale;
- it can promote resilience and mitigate against burnout;
- it has the potential to identify and help to manage clinical problems as well as professional and personal issues;
- it may help with the retention of staff.

Some disadvantages are:

- some clinicians may be reticent to bring issues to a group that could expose their weaknesses or vulnerability;
- there may be the risk of competitiveness between group members;
- not all members of the group may be able to meet due to other demands, e.g. urgent clinical commitments or because of the European working time directive;
- a group with fluid membership may not feel sufficiently safe for some people to raise issues of concern;
- colleagues may collude with each other and find it difficult to be challenging;
- although peer supervision is apparently a relationship between equals there may be power factors, overt and hidden, that make the process less successful;
- some doctors may not value the flat hierarchy of supervision from a peer.

What kind of supervision?

Different models of supervision suit different contexts. Our main experience is in the narrative-based model of exploration (see Chapter 4) that is facilitated by the supervisor asking questions to help the supervisee make a shift in his or her thinking (Halpern

2009). This has been described as 'conversations inviting change' (Launer 2002) and is explained in more detail in Chapter 4. Other forms of supervision are covered in other chapters.

There are many different approaches to thinking about clinical work. Although discussion of cases and issues currently takes place in peer learning groups such as trainers' workshops, this sometimes tends to be discursive when anecdotal experiences are compared and reciprocal advice is offered. Supervisors often have a tendency to speak from their own experience. While this can sometimes be useful, it may not always fit supervisees' contexts or needs and does not help them to develop their own resources or self-supervision skills.

We suggest that a model of supervision, with a formal structure, is more likely to be effective in attending to the particular needs an individual brings. The structure can be readily applied in a variety of situations. It lends itself to being used in peer supervision for doctors as it can address both the technical, developmental and wider pastoral and attitudinal aspects of clinical work. The narrative model is relatively straightforward and the technique can be used to carry out a useful piece of supervision in a timeframe as brief as five to ten minutes. However, the skill in asking questions and picking up relevant cues, and the importance of the careful use of language in supervision is something that requires practice and develops over time. This process happens through observation of others, through receiving feedback oneself and through reflecting on feedback from peers.

How to set up peer supervision

Peer supervision can take place between two colleagues or in a larger group. In a group there will obviously be a wider range of views and observations but attention will also need to be given to managing the group itself. This aspect is dealt with briefly below. We start by considering peer supervision between two colleagues and then move on to ways in which larger groups can operate.

Colleagues may choose to offer each other supervision as a one-off, on an ad hoc basis or as a regular activity. There are pros and cons of having peer supervision with a colleague from the same medical speciality and both should think about whether the advantages of knowing the working context and the ease of access balance the potential disadvantages of familiarity and the risk of making assumptions about the other colleague's options.

The experience of both affirmation and challenge that may come from colleagues within a peer group can promote the value people place both on themselves and others, with a positive impact on personal and professional relationships (Connor and Pakora 2007). This may help clinicians develop skills to survive the stresses of clinical work and to validate and nurture colleagues (Merlevede and Bridoux 2004). An important focus of this kind of work is to reflect on personal interactions within the workplace and on how skills and ideas are applied in everyday practice. This can improve the whole work organization by developing doctors' ability to adapt to change in order to generate new knowledge and continue to improve performance (Fraser and Greenhalgh 2001).

There are a number of ways of working with large groups to carry out peer supervision. The group can be divided into smaller groups consisting of a supervisor, supervisee and observer(s). These groups will work using the same guidelines as for two colleagues and in addition the supervisor or supervisee can indicate that he or she would like to stop at any point to hear comments from others in the group who are observing. This uses the model of a reflecting team (Andersen 1987). When invited to do so, the observers should have a brief conversation with each other while the supervisor and supervisee just listen. The observers may comment on process, for example: 'When X was asked what would happen if she did nothing about the situation, she seemed to become very energized in her response.' They may offer an observation of what has or has not happened, for example: 'It appeared very difficult for the supervisor to get a word in edgeways and ask any questions.' They may also offer some thoughts about questions they would be curious to ask, such as, 'I wonder what X would say if she was asked why she hasn't tackled her trainee about this issue yet.' The supervision then recommences following the lead of where the supervisee wants to take things. The supervisee may or may not wish to respond in the supervision meeting to the comments he or she has heard. Although the observations may have been potentially useful the supervisee may choose to reflect on the comments in private or in a different context.

A larger group can also operate without a specific supervisor, although it may benefit from a group facilitator to keep the group on task, monitor the group dynamics and to act as a safety net. A similar approach has been described by Boscolo and Cecchin (Bertrando and Gilli 2010).

Outline of the method:

1   The facilitator asks group members to give a brief outline of a case that they would like to bring for supervision.
2   The group either chooses a case for supervision within the large group or breaks into smaller groups each considering a different case.
3   Each group listens to the supervisee presenting his or her issue for about five minutes without interruption.
4   The group asks questions to clarify any factual information they think that they need without offering any suggestions or comments.
5   The group discuss their responses for five to ten minutes. The supervisee moves slightly out of the group and just listens to the discussion.
6   The supervisee then says what has been helpful in the group discussion and how he or she will take the case forward.

This method works well with groups who are less experienced in formulating questions. A GP from one group emailed after a session to report:

We tried the format you showed us at the sessional GP group and it worked a treat. There were 13 people present and inevitably some were more assertive than others so when someone offered a case to discuss I suggested we structured the conversation. This meant that everyone participated and the immediate feedback was very positive. I did not introduce it as 'supervision' though mentioned where I had brought it from. I am sure we will use it again when we can maybe discuss the format a little more.

Summary

All doctors in postgraduate training in the UK now need to have supervision. We believe that there are benefits to extending this so that consultants and GPs can continue to participate in supervision as colleagues and peers. Making use of existing learning networks such as those in training schemes and postgraduate education provides a ready-made infrastructure for peer supervision without adversely impacting on time or cost. As we have discussed, peer supervision in the form of professional conversations is already happening. We propose that these conversations can be made more effective by using a structured method that facilitates new ways of thinking. Peer supervision can allow colleagues to bring issues for learning and reflection as well as being a resource for the development of skills through practice and observation throughout professional life.

References

Andersen, T. (1987) The reflecting team: dialogue and meta-dialogue in clinical work, *Family Process*, 26(4): 415–28.

Bertrando, P. and Gilli, G. (2010) Theories of change and the practice of systemic supervision, in C. Burck and G. Daniel (eds) *Mirrors and Reflections: Processes of Systemic Supervision*. London: Karnac Books.

Clutterbuck, D. (2006) *Coaching the Team at Work*. London: Nicholas Brealey International.

Connor, M. and Pakora, J. (2007) *Coaching and Mentoring at Work: Developing Effective Practice*. Maidenhead: McGraw-Hill/Open University Press.

De Kare-Silver, N. (2010) Training for change, *British Journal of General Practice*, DOI: 10.3399/bjgp10X514954.

Fraser, S. and Greenhalgh, T. (2001) Complexity science: coping with complexity, educating for capability, *BMJ*, 323: 799–803.

Halpern, H. (2009) Supervision and the Johari Window: a framework for asking questions, *Education for Primary Care*, 20(1): 10–14.

Kilpatrick, S. (1997) Is there a boundary between formal and non-formal education? The impact of formal and non-formal education on community learning, in *Crossing Borders, Breaking Boundaries: Research in the Education of Adults*. Conference proceedings of 27th annual SCUTREA conference.

Launer, J. (2002) *Narrative-based Primary Care: A Practical Guide*. Oxford: Radcliffe.

Launer, J. (2003) Practice, supervision, consultancy and appraisal: a continuum of learning, *British Journal of General Practice*, 53(493): 662–5.

Merlevede, P. and Bridoux, D. (2004) *Mastering Mentoring and Coaching with Emotional Intelligence*. Bancyfelin, Carmarthen: Crown House Publishing.

Obholzer, A. (1994) Afterword, in A. Obholzer and V. Roberts (eds) *The Unconscious at Work: Individual and Organizational Stress in the Human Services*. London: Routledge.

Shrewsbury, D. and Mohanna, K. (2010) Influencing medical professionalism: innate, taught or caught?, *Education for Primary Care*, 21(3): 199–202.

Taylor, C., Turnbull, C. and Sparrow, N. (2010) Establishing the continuing professional development needs of general practitioners in their first five years after training, *Education for Primary Care*, 21(5): 316–19.

7 Supervision and well-being

Sonya Wallbank

Editors' introduction

In this chapter the author emphasizes how supervision can contribute to well-being and the converse: how lack of it contributes to stress and burnout. She looks at how high expectations of doctors, both their own and other people's, add to their stress – a theme that runs through the book. She describes how attempting to deal with this stress by relying on professional distance is not an effective way of coping with the daily encounter with distress that is part and parcel of a practitioner's life, and how supervision is far more effective. We recognize that for some doctors the impetus to engage in clinical supervision comes from a need to protect their own well-being and for many it is something they look at only once they have lost their well-being. We hope this chapter helps doctors realize the benefits of supervision before they have to pay a high personal price. The writer presents evidence and, as a clinical psychologist who has conducted trials, presents her own experience.

Overview of chapter

This chapter looks at the benefits of supervision as an aid to your well-being, supporting your ability to cope with the demands of your work and restoring your capacity to think clearly. The supervision model described is designed to provide an open space for you to process the emotional demands of your role while challenging you to consider how you impact on others. It encourages you to consider the relationship between your own well-being and that of your patients'. The chapter also provides an overview of quantitative evidence of supervision's value to enable well-being in the workplace, gained with a variety of health professionals including doctors.

Introduction

In this chapter I will focus on supervision as a developmental and supportive process, one which enables cognitive processing of the myriad feelings you, the doctor, are faced with in undertaking your work while allowing your attention to remain focused upon your key tasks. The supervision I describe is designed to draw your attention to aspects of your own performance that could be improved by challenging you to think about those difficult scenarios that you may have struggled with; perhaps areas that have been too difficult for you to think about without a strategy for putting them back in order.

As a clinical psychologist and researcher, I have received some excellent supervision in my professional career. These positive experiences have stayed with me. Supervision has supported my learning; providing a place which I felt was safe enough to enable me to explore aspects of my work self. It has also served as an enabler, a recurrent experience which allows me to focus on aspects of my clinical work which I need to process in more detail, and gives me time to consider my own reaction to work events. As a researcher, I have developed an interest in the quality aspects of supervision, the efficacy of the different models used as well as their utility in supporting professionals. My writing is informed by the supervision I have delivered and evaluated. I have worked with a wide range of different health professionals including doctors and I will also draw on the evidence base of supervision's value to enable well-being in the workplace.

The evidence

I wanted to start the chapter thinking about evidence because I am a great believer in the need to develop an evidence base for the efficacy of such interventions as clinical supervision. I have encountered a myriad of activities given the name 'supervision', not all of which were regarded as beneficial or effective by supervisee or supervisor. This certainly left me with some confusion about what clinical supervision was in different settings and how it was deployed within services. I wanted to begin the chapter by discussing some of the research in which I have been involved that has helped me think about the different types of supervision.

My recent research has enabled me to review the efficacy of restorative supervision, a process which contained elements of psychological support including listening, supporting and challenging supervisees to improve their capacity to cope, especially in difficult and stressful situations. This model allowed the professionals to process their emotional reaction to their work events. It focused on the relationship between supervisees and their colleagues and/or families with whom they work. It is important to recognize that this supervisory process is not therapy. It is primarily focused on workplace events and the impact that these have had upon the professional.

The first study was a randomized controlled trial undertaken with professionals working in obstetrics and gynaecology (Wallbank 2010). It was designed to examine the effectiveness of supervision and found that receiving clinical supervision allowed staff to process their workplace experiences, reducing their scores for burnout, compassion fatigue and subjective stress to non-clinical levels, thus allowing the staff member to be more effective in the workplace. The process also improved compassion satisfaction (the ability of staff members to engage with their patient), which would impact positively on patient care. Anecdotally, staff reported that the process assisted them in improving their own capacity to reflect and cope with their workplace experiences.

A further study undertaken within the West Midlands has looked at the effectiveness of supervision with health visiting and school nurse clinical leaders (Wallbank *et al.* 2010) and has concluded that staff currently experience significant and clinical levels of subjective stress in relation to their work. Although there is no real surprise there for anyone working within the National Health Service (NHS), the study also found that supervisors are likely to be experiencing similar levels of stress and are therefore unable to assist staff in developing more helpful coping strategies or recognizing their distress. This often means individual staff members are on their own: if they are not coping other people may not notice as they could well be overwhelmed themselves.

This has a double effect: not only has collegial support been found to be an important factor in improving individuals' capacity to cope with significant stress but often this is the only appropriate conversation that professionals can have about how they are feeling. The less opportunity there is to have collegial conversation, the more need there is to find other (less effective perhaps) ways of coping. Post-supervision measures showed a significant reduction in burnout and stress and demonstrated how supervision supported the complex nature of the safeguarding work undertaken by professionals. They reported being clearer about risk factors and caseload management and felt more confident to undertake the work. The supervision process appeared to enable professionals to think and allowed learning to be generalized, encouraging appropriate action when professionals were faced with their next complex situation (Wallbank 2010).

Supervision that increases our ability to cope

One of the most significant pieces of comparative data that has remained consistent across the studies I have led is that the levels of distress experienced by NHS staff working in areas such as obstetrics and gynaceology and safeguarding are significantly worse than similar studies undertaken with police, army and ambulance staff who were reflecting on working with death and dying (Joseph 2000).

If the impact of the work is ignored and professionals feel unsupported within their role by management or through the absence of explicit and available support systems, the more likely they are to give up their career. The NHS loses experienced and skilled professionals every day because they are just unable to carry on with the status quo (Unite/CPHVA 2007).

Supervision in varying forms has been shown to be effective in increasing staff job satisfaction, reducing stress and burnout and improving quality of care (Hyrkas *et al.* 2006; Wallbank 2010). Where staff are experiencing high levels of stress, they are likely to feel overwhelmed by their workload and will have a reduced decision-making capacity. Increasing coping skills will have a positive impact on patient care as the practitioner is more likely to be able to consider the wider needs of patients and their families. Families who need support in changing detrimental health behaviours require professionals who are emotionally available and engaged with the family's needs. This requires an effort on the part of the health professional, which supervision aims to support. The following is an example of how supervision can support the capacity of professionals to be able to think about their own behaviour.

CASE EXAMPLE: MICHELLE

Michelle had been recently promoted to Clinical Lead when she began supervision sessions. She was finding the increased clinical and managerial demands difficult and appeared to have inherited some difficult team dynamics within her clinical team. During her first sessions, Michelle struck me as being unable to think; she had rigid ideas about what her colleagues' motivations might be towards her and was very negative about possible alternative explanations of her staff's behaviours. Michelle went on to discuss her uncertainty about taking the role and how she believed others felt she was less experienced than she should have been to get offered the role. She seemed to interpret others' input as a threat to her own credibility. We began to think about the way Michelle may be projecting a lack of certainty onto the team and that this might be resulting in some anxious behaviour from the team. Michelle began to consider over the next few sessions how she needed to see herself as a leader before others could take her seriously. As her behaviour changed so did that of others towards her and she became more confident. Dealing with the pressing issues in a practical way freed her up to think creatively and she continued to develop strongly.

This example serves to remind us that how we behave affects how people behave towards us. Often our work persona is not challenged in the same way that it would be in our home life, as our colleagues may feel unable to tell us things that are 'difficult' to talk about. When we behave in difficult ways it takes someone to complain about us before we can see our own influence. Supervision is often a mirror which allows us to see enough of ourselves to make a difference without the threat of others telling us what we need to do. The supervisor does not have all the answers but often knows the questions that are difficult to ask. These might be questions around why you have decided on a particular course of action; challenging your reaction especially where your behaviour has been difficult or avoidant and attempting to connect you to experiences you may have preferred not to think about. The process can raise your consciousness about issues that you may have known were there but were unable to reflect on independently. It supports the process of managing the natural anxiety that working in a stressful environment creates and enables us to develop positive models of leadership. It also allows us to identify and break patterns of behaviour that may have reduced our effectiveness previously and can support our ability to influence people and build relationships as we remain aware of the reciprocal nature of relationships. I think supervision also enables us to recognize the signs of stress in others and means that we are functioning at a level that enables us to offer support.

Having to cope

I often wonder what an alien would make of looking in on the world of a doctor. All the usual caveats as to what an individual should expect to experience as 'normal' are removed. These are replaced by the familiar and consistent experience of human misery, pain, loss, despair and devastation, to name a few. Why is it that we have such high expectations of doctors – that whatever they are faced with, professionalism will be enough to see them through?

When faced with extraordinary events, humans have an amazing capacity to adapt. It is both useful and essential for doctors to keep a clear head and have enough clarity of thought to be able to make rational decisions which impact on patients and their families. Do the strategies needed to achieve this distance compromise patient care? Is this useful in shielding professionals from the reality of the decisions they are making?

Perhaps those who do not develop such strategies, identifying with the patient and/or the patient's family, quickly become burnt out and stressed from the emotional burden they are forced to carry. The idea that trauma and tragedy can be experienced on a regular basis without negative side effects is certainly not empirically sound. When professionals do become hardened to their experiences, is this when patient care suffers? I wonder what sort of doctor you would like to have as a patient yourself? One who is technically superior but emotional burnt out or one who has managed to engage with the complexities of a doctor's work and retain his or her humanity? Perhaps doctors who are given the opportunity to process their experiences are more likely to continue case holding or working directly with patients for longer – an interesting idea for a longitudinal study.

Recognizing the need to process what happens to you

CASE EXAMPLE: MALCOLM

Malcolm was a senior consultant, and well regarded in his workplace. He was used to dealing with loss and described himself as much more comfortable delivering bad news than hearing it. Within a few minutes of entering the room we had designated for supervision, he began to tell me how he had wanted to reschedule the session. He had not really seen the need for supervision but felt he might as well see me anyway. A few minutes later, after agreeing some ground rules and how the confidentiality of the sessions would work, Malcolm began to tell me about John, a father, not his own but a patient whom he had met ten years earlier. Being a more junior member of staff back then he was able to spend more time with this patient and his family.

The downside was that he watched and experienced the family's distress as John did not survive.

Malcolm recalled with minute detail how he heard that John had died and how he was unable to talk to anyone about it. Unfortunately he had been on leave for a few days following the loss and did not have any opportunity for an informal debrief with his colleagues. Instead he had remained at home, alone, and continued to think about the failings of his own profession. Years later, Malcolm had still not come to terms with the loss and carried this around like a dead weight. As he recalled John and his feelings at this time, Malcolm became extremely distressed and although this passed quickly he was visibly shocked by his own response. He was quickly able to regain his usual professional stance but looked visibly lighter.

Malcolm used subsequent sessions as an opportunity to think about his own actions and the inevitability of the loss. John had been diagnosed with a terminal condition prior to being admitted to Malcolm's care. This had been a difficult diagnosis for John and his family to come to terms with. They appeared to be holding out the hope that a miracle cure or explanation would come along. When Malcolm took over John's care he became burdened with this sense of responsibility that the family seemed to project onto him. He developed a close relationship with John and his family and recalled powerful feelings of helplessness as John's condition worsened. During supervision Malcolm was able to understand how the powerful feelings that John and his family were experiencing may have impacted on him. This was his first experience of providing palliative care for a patient and one that appeared at odds with Malcolm's desire to help people through medicine. Feeling that he was unable to offer any solace to John or his family left him with an overwhelming sense of responsibility. The sessions enabled Malcolm to process this experience and think about how he might have dealt with the situation differently. Rather than discuss the impact of John's death on him, Malcolm became withdrawn and eventually was signed off sick. He spent a long period of time on his own thinking about how his choice of career was misguided. Identifying that he was inexperienced and would have benefited from talking to someone about how he was feeling allowed Malcolm to normalize what had happened. He was able to file it away as a natural part of his career – but just one that needed to be processed.

I imagine that Malcolm's experience of losing a patient whom he had got to know is ubiquitous across the medical profession, especially in early training. What was significant to Malcolm was the level of responsibility he had accepted for this loss. He had retained a skewed recollection of events, only remembering the distress and sadness rather than the reassurances of his colleagues and supervisors at the time. Unfortunately, working within a profession which has high expectations of how one reacts to emotional events, this was not talked about or discussed. Malcolm was unable to take the difficulties he was having home to family or friends or to discuss and share his experiences. Instead, he recalled how every loss felt as though he was revisiting this event. He was unable to file this experience away and it certainly felt as if he had not processed the event.

The model of restorative supervision most familiar to me involves critical reflection and developing a sense of understanding of why you have behaved in a particular way. It enables you to remain aware of your patients and their holistic needs as well as to learn lessons from your experiences. This understanding can then be used to influence how you cope with the stress of the role and support the development of more positive ways of behaving.

For Malcolm, despite the passage of time, John was still on his mind. Traumatic experiences which have not been processed (thought about and digested to allow you to make sense of them) tend to stick out in your mind and are often revisited or intrude on your day-to-day thoughts. This would have impacted on John's ability to process subsequent patient loss and influence his decision-making skills. Supervision allowed John to think about the events constructively and experience the distress (which is often the reason individuals avoid thinking about events that were traumatic). The distress quickly passed and Malcolm could think with another person about how the events played out and why they remained so significant for him. This allowed Malcolm to file the event away and literally remove them from his working memory. This would have impacted positively on his emotional well-being as he no longer needed to attend to the consistent thoughts and negative feelings he was experiencing.

Carrying and acting out the burdens

The stress of doctors has already been recognized and discussed earlier in this book. Understanding why events may be perceived as stressful and what you subsequently do to support yourself with this stress is crucial to making you more resilient. Your coping style has been recognized as mediating the effects that stress can have on you (Lazarus and Folkman 1984). Certain coping styles such as avoidance (not talking about it; trying not to think about it) or venting (becoming agitated or angry with others about the stressor or an unrelated matter to disperse your feelings) have been shown to significantly increase the impact of stress. As a doctor you may be reluctant to immerse yourself in talking with others about your vulnerabilities and this in itself means you are more likely to opt for negative ways of coping.

It may be that the way you process events is different. For some people, running or physical fitness allows them the mental space to think about how their day has unfolded. For others, a quick drink and some black humour with colleagues is enough to allow them to manage the cognitive demands of the role. The difficulty is that these strategies may not be enough when something goes wrong or an event is perceived by you to be more traumatic than other events. Suppressing events can in itself lead to you experiencing them in more intense or frequent form later. If you have tried purposefully not to think about something, it often ends up being the only thing that your mind can attend to.

Recognizing the need for others

The process of verbalizing your feelings and allowing yourself time and opportunity to experience what has happened to you is essential for reducing the impact of the events. This is why 'emotional literacy' has become so important in recent years as we have learnt that children who can talk about how they feel are much more resilient even in the face of very difficult circumstances (Rudd 2009).

Social support is seen as the single most protective factor in a myriad of difficult circumstances (Regehr and Bober 2005) but for doctors who are covered by patient confidentiality and a need to protect their family from the distress they have experienced, sharing the day over a glass of wine or home-cooked meal is not healthy – for the relationship or the professionalism of the doctor. Faced with partners who are unable to talk, relationships can often suffer as the other person feels uninvolved and unable to help. It becomes more difficult to suppress how you are feeling, behaviour changes, agitation increases and the negative impact is felt by those closest to you. Here is one example of how significant events that are not processed can sometimes 'spill out' despite your best efforts.

CASE EXAMPLE: TONY

We were having dinner with friends, both consultants in different medical specialities. After a couple of drinks Tony began to tell us about his dreadful day. This was strange as Tony never talked about work. It sounded as though there had been an awful set of unanticipated events which had resulted in the loss of a newborn baby. Tony was the doctor responsible for the delivery and he had needed to remain strong to cope with the understandable impact of the events on the family and his team of staff. The difficulty was that Tony had also experienced these events as distressing and it seemed to challenge his assumptions about the way he had carried out his work. He had not felt it appropriate to display visibly within this workplace how he was feeling and he described how at one point he nearly cried, he was so ashamed that he might let the family and his staff down in this way. Sarah, his wife, looked horrified as Tony became more upset and appeared very keen to move the conversation on. The next day, we received a frantic call from Sarah apologizing for Tony and asking us to respect that this could be a high-profile loss and we should not mention it to anyone.

Tony had clearly not meant to say anything that night but perhaps the wine or the fact that he was clearly overwhelmed by the events led him to an unusual need to share his emotions. I was left wondering which was worse: that he had to experience such moving events or that they both felt so ashamed of their lack of control of their emotions surrounding the events. Often clinical supervision can be the ideal place to be able to share such significant events and process your reaction to them without the risk of being judged or needing to remain completely in control of your emotional reactions. Our families or friends are often the first in line to catch our work life experiences as they leak out often when we don't intend them to do so. Often people are unprepared or unable to give us the responses we need at this point and we can feel worse for sharing this information. Supervision would have enabled Tony to recognize the intense experience he had been subjected to. He would have been able to think about his own actions or reactions and gain some insight into how the events would feature in his subsequent decision making. This would mean that in the future when faced with subsequent experiences he could remain assured in his decision making and not burdened with the loss he was unable to alter.

Doctors' well-being transfers to patients

Recognition of individuals working within the NHS and their emotional needs appears current thinking as the modernization of the NHS continues to move forward. The link between doctors who are content and happy within their work and positive patient care is not a difficult one to make.

> Staff satisfaction and levels of engagement can be improved if organizations ensure that the importance of their staff's health and well-being are recognized . . . and where there are clear benefits, providing early intervention services.
>
> (DH 2009a)

What is not so easy is the appropriate response for the individual. Often interventions have little or no empirical evidence attached to them and are underutilized by those they are meant to support. Occupational health has been set up for years to be able to respond to staff in distress but this model fails to recognize that often the distress is a normal part of dealing with this work and should be treated as such. The preferred model of staff dysfunction where the individual needs to seek out the most appropriate treatment means that individuals prefer not to self-refer as they worry that this will mean they are labelled as dysfunctional.

Supervision should be seen as an inoculation and early intervention, with preventative benefits for being able to cope with the most difficult aspects of our work. It helps you protect yourself from the distress that is all around the workplace and share in confidence what the impact was for you individually without feeling the need to be judged or your performance measured in some way. It is not a remedial or corrective process but one which enables well-being, coping and the capacity to think and feel clearly.

Summary

This chapter has looked at how the expectations of doctors to cope with the content of their work can have a detrimental impact on their ability to process their experiences. Consistent exposure to trauma and human distress lies outside of the usual human experience and needs to be processed as such. The usual support systems of the individual doctor have been discussed. These may not be available given the content of the work and the need to protect the confidentiality of the patient and the doctor's family from experiencing the distress of the professional. An empirical case for supervision has been presented which describes some of the positive results of supervision studies and the aspects of well-being on which supervision is seen to have an impact. Safeguarding has been used as one aspect of practice that creates a great deal of anxiety and supervision is seen to be of benefit here. Finally, the chapter has reflected on ways of thinking and how these might be improved as well as looking at current levels of staff stress.

References

DH (Department of Health) (2009a) *NHS Health and Well-being: The Boorman Review*. London: Department of Health.

Hyrkas, K., Appelqvist-Schmidlechner, K. and Haataja, R. (2006) Efficacy of clinical supervision: influence on job satisfaction, burnout and quality of care, *Journal of Advanced Nursing*, 55(4): 521–35.

Joseph, S. (2000) Psychometric evaluation of Horowitz's impact of events scale: a review, *Journal of Traumatic Stress*, 13: 101–13.

Lazarus, R. S. and Folkman, S. (1984) *Stress, Appraisal and Coping*. Oxford: Springer Publishing.

Regehr, C. and Bober, T. (2005) *In the Line of Fire: Trauma in the Emergency Services*. Oxford: Oxford University Press.

Rudd, B. (ed.) (2009) *Help Your Child Develop Emotional Literacy: A Parent's Guide to Happy Children*. London: Network Continuum Education.

Unite/CPHVA (Community Practitioners' and Health Visitors' Association) (2007) *Community Practitioners' and Health Visitors' Association Response to 'Facing the Future: A Review of the Role of Health Visitors'*. London: Unite/CPHVA.

Wallbank, S. (2010) Effectiveness of individual clinical supervision for midwives and doctors in stress reduction, *Evidence Based Midwifery*, 8(2): 28–34.

Wallbank, S., McKeown, C., Jones, L. and Hawkes, J. (2010) *Safeguarding Children Care Pathway Report*. Birmingham: NHS West Midlands.

8   Coaching for doctors

Anita Houghton

Editors' introduction

Coaching is being used increasingly in the NHS and we wanted to include it in this book on supervision partly because there are many overlaps with supervision and partly because we want to support anything that can safely and effectively contribute to the well-being of doctors. Both this chapter and the previous one place a strong emphasis on this self-care and while this is desirable in its own right it is also a prerequisite for the sustainable care of patients. Much of the philosophy underpinning both coaching and supervision are shared. Many of the techniques, resources and practices of one, can and do contribute to the 'tool kit' of the other. As editors we are interested in both the many similarities and the differences, actual and perceived, between supervision and coaching. Some techniques, like using good questions (see Chapter 4) and letting the coachee/supervisee determine aspects of the agenda, have been described in earlier chapters. As editors we are aware and interested that there is some lack of clarity in many users and providers about the difference between supervision and coaching. We notice that coaching often has more of an emphasis on the performance and/or the career of the coachee, often over a short but focused period of time, whereas clinical supervision is more likely to focus on situations that involve patients and a supervisee's personal development, often with a longer-term perspective. Both involve looking at old situations in new ways to enhance how an individual works while sustaining his or her well-being.

Overview of chapter

This chapter is about doctors and coaching. It talks first about the nature of medicine, its culture and the kinds of people who tend to become doctors. It goes on to talk of how these things can combine to produce problems in the workplace, problems that can be both prevented and ameliorated through coaching. By the end of it the reader should understand what coaching is, the kinds of work issues that it can be useful for, what typically happens in a coaching session, and some idea of the techniques that are used.

Introduction

A few years ago, when I had responsibility for arranging part-time training for junior doctors, a young trainee approached me. At the time she was doing a very busy neurology job at a London teaching hospital. As well as a heavy on-call commitment she was finding it difficult to leave the hospital before 8 or 9 in the evening on normal days. At home she had a husband and two young children. By the time she arrived home the children were in bed, which was just as well because she then had to start work on writing up her PhD thesis. It is more or less impossible to progress in neurology without a PhD or equivalent.

Unsurprisingly this exhausting schedule was beginning to take its toll and she looked worn out and anxious. She had come to me to ask if she could work part-time. I asked her if she had spoken to anybody at work about the hours she was having to work. She said that she had been reluctant to do that in case she was seen as 'not consultant material' and that that would damage her prospects. She had become so desperate that she had in fact gathered herself up to approach her consultant the previous week. She'd managed to catch him at the end of a ward round and had explained to him that she was finding it difficult to manage all her commitments and that her hours at work meant that she was having to work on her thesis late at night and into the early hours. His jovial reply had been, 'Oh I always say that the best work is done after midnight!' followed by a wink and, 'You've got to be seen as robust, you know.' And off he went.

That one story encapsulates so much of what being a junior doctor in the NHS can be like. A widespread feature is that you almost always have too much to do for the hours that you are employed to work. The result is that you are stressed, tired and unlikely to be at your most efficient or effective self. That produces more stress, more inefficiency and an increased risk of making mistakes. Within your working time you are dealing with the suffering and anxiety and sadness of your patients and their families, which, too, absorbs a great deal of your energy. As a junior you are also learning and so are regularly faced with clinical situations that are outside your experience and competence. Because you can't do everything within working hours, your personal life becomes eroded to the stage when you can barely remember what your partner looks like, let alone your friends. Even when you do manage to get home you either have exams to study for, or theses or papers to write. If you don't have any of these, you spend your time worrying about events during the day. Did I take care of that patient properly? Was I a bit short-tempered with that nurse? Oh no, I forgot to do the blood test on that patient. You are too frightened to talk to anyone, either peers or consultants, because the culture states that you must be seen to be coping. You worry that any sign of weakness could generate doubts about your suitability for the job, and even as you're considering asking for support you can imagine a darkened room where grave faces pore over your appraisal documents and heads are shaken sadly. So you keep quiet. You feel ashamed at your dismal capacity to cope, and because you never talk to anyone you assume that you are the only doctor in the hospital, and quite possibly the world, that is struggling.

If you get through this period in your career, and not everyone does, you become a consultant or a GP, and while you tend to have more control over your time than as a junior, the idea of not coping or asking for help becomes even more taboo. The slightest sign of self-doubt is likely to strike fear into the heart of your clinical director or GP partner and result in the kind of close vigilance that few could survive.

When passing from junior to senior roles, as well as suddenly finding yourself 'where the buck stops' in your clinical work, you discover that you have all kinds of other responsibilities for which you've received absolutely no training. You have a secretary to manage and make best use of. You have clinics or surgeries to organize. You have juniors to supervise, multidisciplinary colleagues to rub along with and a team to lead. Then you discover that if you want increments on your salary or a clinical excellence award, performing your clinical duties alone is not enough. You need to do research, reorganize your department, take a managerial post, become involved in postgraduate training, speak at conferences. And most of this you will have to do alone.

The nature of the beast

Added to the 'must be seen to cope' culture are the psychological mindsets that are common to doctors. First and foremost is the drive to succeed. Bright children at school theoretically have more choice of careers than less bright ones but, paradoxically, in practice they don't. When a young person does well in exams their parents, teachers and society at large immediately start forming expectations about them. And what do they expect of them? That they will pursue one of the top careers. It isn't difficult to guess what comes at the top of their list of prestigious careers. Medicine. Or perhaps law. Or accountancy. Or The City.

So doctors tend to come from a background of Great Expectations, and when their parents and teachers are no longer putting pressure on them to succeed they naturally take on that role for themselves. The result is often perfectionism and a high degree of self-criticism, both of which are risk factors for stress and depression. For perfectionists, anything that falls short of perfection is a failure. There is no in-between. When a mistake is made, however small, perfectionists will give themselves a severe beating that may last for days or even weeks. Although used to success after success, the further doctors go in their career, the more likely they are to face failure of some sort. A first failed exam, an unsuccessful interview, a clinical case that went wrong, a complaint from a patient, a troublesome relationship with a colleague. What may seem like mere hiccoughs to other people can feel catastrophic to a perfectionist.

The ego of people whose identity rests on success is therefore often fragile, and they will go to extraordinary lengths to avoid failure. Hence the atmospheres of medical institutions are often highly competitive, and the more prestigious the institution the more competitive the culture. Somebody who believes their very existence depends on ostentatious success may be charming and supportive when things are going well, but when they are under threat they are capable of doing whatever is necessary to defend themselves and their territory. It is therefore not surprising that bullying is commonly reported by doctors. In a survey of a thousand BMA members in 2002, 37 per cent said they had been bullied during the last year (a definition was supplied), and 84 per cent reported having been at the receiving end of one or more behaviours that appear on a validated bullying scale (Quine 2002). There is also corroborating evidence from the annual NHS staff survey.

Doctors are chosen primarily for their academic ability. That means that while they are being selected for their exam results they are, by default, being selected for their personality traits. Doctors tend to be conscientious, for example, and are often organized and reliable. They also tend to be rationalists, scientists who are good at analysing a situation objectively and making decisions based on logic and cause and effect.

Doctors, however, are a varied breed. The type described above may be prevalent and instantly recognizable, but there are other types within the medical workforce. Some will go into medicine because they are passionate about science and the human body. Some go into medicine because they want to care for people. Some want a career which is secure and where they won't have to fight for jobs or recognition because the career structure is clear and progressive. Many go into medicine because it pays better than almost any other profession, and because there is a status in being a doctor. Some will go into medicine for all of these reasons; others for only one or two.

The personality types who are in the majority within the profession or a speciality, however, tend to create the culture, and the atmosphere they create tends to attract people who are just like them. The culture is therefore self-perpetuating and can be very uncomfortable for those that don't fit in. Culture varies from one speciality to another, but in general the kinds of people who fit in are rational, organized, practical, assertive and somewhat detached. The types who find it more difficult to fit in are intuitive, creative, easy-going, sensitive and people-oriented. These people are especially in need of the kind of support that supervision and coaching can provide.

The health and well-being of doctors

Jenny Firth-Cozens became well known in medical circles for her longitudinal study, starting in 1983, of the mental health of a cohort of medical students (Firth-Cozens 1999). The study was stimulated by a question that two registrars asked her. Two of their house officers had committed suicide; everybody was shocked and upset, and yet nobody talked about it – it was unmentionable. Could somebody do something, they asked, about the stress and depression that they saw around them? In an editorial in the *BMJ* (Firth-Cozens 2003) she takes a look at what has changed, and what has not, over the years since she started that study. One thing that has not changed is that around 28 per cent of doctors consistently report above threshold levels of stress and other psychological morbidity, compared to 18 per cent of the general working population (Wall *et al.* 1997). Key work factors associated with psychological ill health and sickness absence are long hours worked, work overload and pressure, and the effects of these on personal lives; lack of control over work; lack of participation in decision making; poor social support; and unclear management and work role.

Another factor that has been consistently reported is that female doctors are more likely to experience stress and burnout than men. A study of the psychological type of doctors, and its relation to job satisfaction, may provide a clue (G. Clack, personal communication). Jungian typology, which can be measured using the Myers-Briggs Type Indicator, distinguishes between people who prefer to make decisions based on objective analysis (thinking deciders) and those who prefer to make decisions based on personal values and the effect on people (feeling deciders) (Myers and McCaulley 1985). Clack discovered that job satisfaction was lower in feeling deciders. As around 66 per cent of women are feeling deciders whereas around 66 per cent of men are thinking deciders, it could be that because women are more likely to be empathic and compassionate types they are more vulnerable to stress and burnout. That may be because they are inherently more vulnerable, or because they have to work in a culture that is antipathetical to those qualities.

What has changed?

What has changed, says Firth-Cozens (2003), is the acceptance that stress is an issue, for patients, individual staff and the organizations they work for:

> Contrary to the experience of the two registrars, doctors have become used to discussing the topic of stress and even to admitting to it in themselves. They are more aware of their colleagues' symptoms than they were, which means that they may be more likely to help colleagues through a difficult time or suggest they get help when they need it.

She goes on to say that, furthermore, organizations have finally accepted that stress costs them vast amounts of money – through absence, litigation, and the fact that unhappy, tense, tired or anxious doctors do not produce quality care (Firth-Cozens 2001). It has been shown that stressed doctors are at higher risk of making mistakes, particularly if they are short of sleep (Jones *et al.* 1988; Weinger and Ebden 2002). However, we now know that lack of sleep and other stressors can be ameliorated if a doctor has good support. Supportive teams, for example, have less stressed staff (Carter and West 1999).

Firth-Cozens, in her paper, notes that much has improved since she first started her study. Hours have reduced, training has improved, and a number of support agencies have been set up, such as the National Sick Doctors' association, the BMA's Doctors for Doctors services and employee support schemes at work. She then says:

> However, I am not aware that a truly proactive means of attending to the health of NHS staff, including doctors, has been planned.
>
> (Firth-Cozens 2003)

What kinds of needs do doctors have?

In my experience as a doctors' coach, the kinds of issues that crop up tend to fall into one or more of the following categories:

- Career problems: early when making decisions, later when chosen pathway is not working out, later still when in a rut and looking for new challenges, or wanting to wind down to retirement.
- Transition from junior to consultant – increased clinical responsibility, new managerial/administrative responsibilities, sudden reduction in support.
- Patients and relatives we find difficult, adverse events, patient suicides, mistakes, complaints.
- Taking more senior roles that require strategic and people management skills, and that change and sometimes rupture relationships with colleagues.
- Performance problems: clinical competence, disciplinary action, errors, underperformance, referral to the National Clinical Assessment Service or the General Medical Council.
- Personal difficulties: mental or physical ill health, stress, not coping, addictions, problems with colleagues, problems in personal life.

On a personal level, doctors need help in:

- forming realistic expectations of themselves;
- accepting the feelings that some situations and patients produce in them;
- having a life outside work;
- solving problems;
- learning skills they need for their non-clinical responsibilities;
- coping with unreasonable and stressful workloads;
- handling change and transition;
- looking after their health;
- developing themselves as individuals;
- keeping their skills and knowledge up to date;
- understanding the system in which they work;
- getting along with their colleagues;
- managing their juniors and other staff

and perhaps most importantly:

- including themselves among the people they look after.

Coaching can help doctors explore and learn from all these areas, but unfortunately doctors are often reluctant to seek help. My experience of coaching the profession has taught me that doctors are intelligent, conscientious, self-reliant, committed to doing their best, driven to succeed, and have great mental and physical stamina. When the volume of these admirable attributes is turned up too high, however, the other qualities that doctors require to manage their own needs are ignored, they are often reluctant to admit they need help, and even more reluctant to seek it. The result is that by the time doctors ask for help they are often in a bad way. The secret of developing a medical workforce that is healthy, happy, and can therefore provide optimum care for their patients, is to view support as an ongoing need, not something that you seek only when you're on your knees.

How can coaching help?

The aim of coaching is, very simply, to help people feel better today, and to move towards the kind of future they would like. It can be applied to just about any part of life. The underlying assumption is that individuals have all the resources they need to solve their problems, and it is the coach's job to help them to find these resources. The philosophy behind coaching is that the relationship between coach and coachee is essentially equal and the two work closely together.

A fascinating feature of coaching is that a coach can help a client with a problem while knowing very little about the technical or specific aspects of the problem. For this reason, coaches are trained to keep out of the 'content' of the client's story, and just apply the techniques. To illustrate, in one of the final assessments of my Masters course we were asked to coach another participant through a problem which that person was only allowed to relate symbolically. For example, the 'client' might say: 'I've got a green in my life who doesn't blue enough, and that makes me pink.' The coach would then have to use his or her skills to help the person more forward with that problem. Hard though it is to believe, the clients repeatedly reported new insights and solutions to their problem, despite the coach knowing almost nothing about it. That is the extraordinary power of good quality coaching.

This approach could scarcely be more different from that of many doctors. Doctors are trained to listen to their patients, work out what is wrong with them and then tell them what they can do about it. In coaching the assumption is that the only expert in the room is the client. Nobody can know the story better than the client, nobody can understand it better, and therefore nobody can know quite as well as that person what will and won't work in terms of a solution.

What happens in a coaching session?

Doctors come to coaching for a variety of reasons and via a variety of routes. Many make a private decision to seek help. Others are offered individual or group coaching as part of a management course. Some are offered coaching because their manager or director recognizes the need for support and development in their role and wants to offer them that opportunity; others are referred because there are problems with their performance.

Whatever the reason, and whatever the route, an initial session with a coach will tend to revolve around the following questions:

- Tell me about yourself and what has brought you to coaching? (Example: I'm a registrar in dermatology and I'm unhappy in my job.)
- What would you like to get from coaching? (Example: I'd like to understand better what is going wrong for me in this job/speciality, to decide whether I want to stay in it, and if not, what I want to do instead.)
- If the coaching was successful, what would you have at the end of it that is different to now? (Example: I would know more about what has gone wrong, have a decision about a way forward, and have a plan.)

It would be rare for someone to be that clear about what they wanted until well into the first session. Most doctors who come to me have never in their lives before had an hour of a professional's time to themselves that is client-led. The very act of talking through a situation, which has probably been preoccupying them for many of their waking hours, and for many months, can be extraordinarily liberating and helpful. Nevertheless, while providing an open space for talking and reflection, you can see from the questions that guide the first session that coaching tends to have direction.

Another feature of coaching, which differs from some other forms of supervision, is that there is an emphasis on taking action between sessions. This action might be to read a particular book, have a conversation with someone, tidy the office, do a coaching exercise, and so on. The premise, again, is that the client is the expert in his or her problem, and is also the only person who can put it right. Often doctors have been struggling with a situation for some time and have tried a variety of ways of putting it right. The reason they have come to see you is that none of them have worked. A coaching session can help to review what they've been doing, understand why it hasn't been working and consider what else they can try. As Einstein said, 'You can't solve a problem with the same thinking that caused it.' Coaching helps a person to have new perspectives on old problems, and so find new ways forward.

While most doctors seek coaching to solve particular problems, some will do so because they want to perform better at work generally, progress their career, or develop certain skills. It's therefore often appropriate to split time between tackling current challenges and developing more generally. Doctors who come to coaching over a period of time will start to notice major differences in how they handle themselves and their experience of life. A coach may suggest, for example, exploring your psychological type, so that you can both shed light on current difficulties and increase your understanding of your natural strengths and possible blind spots, and how they differ from other people's. She might suggest exploring what is important to you at work, what motivates and demotivates you. She will help you to build emotional intelligence, interpersonal skills, organizational skills, and to explore ways in which you can develop professionally. She may help you to look at how you balance your time, both within work, and between work and personal life.

When somebody is planning to have regular coaching I will usually start by asking them to work through some questions and exercises that help them to take an overview of their working lives. An exercise used by many coaches is the 'Wheel of Life' (see below).

The Wheel of Life

Take a piece of paper and write down all the roles you play in your life, for example doctor, parent, spouse, householder, financial manager, friend. When you have done that, write down your seven main roles in life, combining some of your roles if necessary. For example, you might combine son/daughter, aunt/uncle/ brother/sister into 'family member'.

When you have the seven main roles, write the roles on the spokes of the wheel below, adding 'self-carer' to the eighth spoke. Doctors invariably neglect this one, but it is the most important of all – your well-being and development affects the way you play every other role. You play this role when you are developing yourself, relaxing, doing things you enjoy, and looking after your health, your spiritual development, and your general well-being.

Then do the following:

- Rate your current level of satisfaction with each role, where 0 is low satisfaction and 10 is high, and make a dot on the line at the appropriate point. Label these dots 'PS' for 'present satisfaction'.
- Now place a second mark on each line at the point which reflects where you would like your score to be in that particular role. Label these 'DS' for 'desired satisfaction'.
- Join the PS dots to gain a visual image of your current state of balance, then join the DS dots.

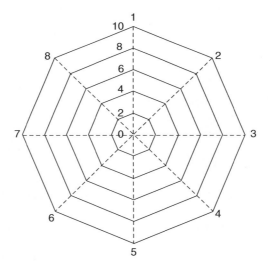

Looking at your wheel, ask yourself:

- What do these results mean to me?
- What do I see in this overview of my life, in terms of satisfaction and balance?

- Is there anything missing that should be there?
- In which role am I performing the least? The best?
- Where are the greatest gaps between present and desired satisfaction?
- What do I need or want to change first?

Imagine you had a performance rating of 10 for every role. How would you be acting/behaving? What results would you see? What would relationships be like?

Finally, if you were to choose the one role to work on that would make the most difference to your life, which would it be? Set yourself three small actions for that role.

Because most doctors have not been to a coach before it is important to explain what they can expect from the process, and what is expected of them. Many coaches will have some form of contract or agreement, and I have given an example of such an agreement below.

A coaching agreement

This agreement lays out what you can expect of me, your coach, and what you are committing yourself to as the client.

What you can expect from me:
- I am here to listen to you, to help you to develop and move forward in your life, and to support you in tackling specific issues.
- I shall treat the content of our sessions as strictly confidential.
- I will normally divide the time between helping you to develop generally, and helping you to deal with specific challenges. The balance between these, and what we work on, will always be with your agreement.
- I may ask you to do strange things!
- I will often suggest activities for you to do between sessions.
- I'll be available by email for emergencies between sessions.

My requests of you are, please:
- to be as open as you can;
- to be prepared to try new things;
- to tell me if there is anything you would like to change about the sessions, or anything you are unhappy with;
- to commit to getting the most from coaching;
- to set aside time between sessions to do the suggested activities.

Group coaching

Sometimes coaching is offered in groups, variously known as learning sets, action learning sets, or development sets. These are often set up to support particular groups of people. Chief Executives, Medical Directors and Directors of Public Health, for example, will often belong to a group of this kind, and will meet every few weeks or months. Some GPs form groups like these as well. These groups can go on for several years, while others are more short-term. The King's Fund in London, for example, uses development sets as an integral part of their management courses for doctors, a half day set aside for this activity in each module. Sometimes these groups will continue meeting once the course has finished but often they just meet three or four times.

There are different ways of running groups like this. Most will be facilitated, at least to start with, and the facilitator may use part of the time to teach self-management techniques, such as communication exercises, time management, exploring values, and so on. Time will also be spent on helping the group to bond and get to know each other. But at the core of all these groups will be a focus on individual issues and a space for exploring these with the help of the other members. A common method is very similar to that of Balint groups (see Chapter 3), in which an individual (the 'client') will be given fifty minutes to an hour to explore a particular issue. Typically that person will be given some uninterrrupted time, first of all, to describe the situation or problem that he or she is dealing with. Members of the group will then ask questions of clarification for a few minutes, before going on to questions aimed at helping the person understand the situation better, gain new perspectives on it and find ways forward. As with Balint groups, towards the latter stages the person is invited to turn away from the group, while still listening, whereupon the other members will then reflect on the issue and, if they wish, offer solutions. An important rule is that suggestions and advice are not allowed during question time. Doctors find this almost unbearable as they are so used to offering solutions and their whole identity often rests on their ability to do so. Some people almost need physical restraint to stop them from leaping in with their advice!

There's an important reason for not allowing advice or suggestions to be directed at the client and it relates to the premise that it is the client who has the solution to his or her problems, not the coach. If you have ever been in a situation with someone who is in difficulty (other than a patient) you will probably have experienced this reason first hand. Let's say a medical friend is having trouble with a colleague at work. 'Why don't you speak to your consultant about it?', you say, helpfully. 'Well, I thought of that,' he says, 'but she is friends with this person and I don't think she would back me.' 'So why don't you go to the clinical director then?' 'I've thought of that too,' he says, 'but the clinical director is really stressed out at the moment over a department reorganization, and he's not going to want to hear about this.' 'But surely,' you say, 'it's his responsibility to deal with this?' 'Well yes,' he says, 'but the reality is...'

There are at least two undesirable results of this kind of conversation. First and foremost is that the conversation is unhelpful to the client. Secondly, it disrupts the relationship between the two of you because you become increasingly frustrated and he becomes increasingly defensive. Once that happens a positive outcome is unlikely.

This is one of the reasons why we set aside time for people to give their suggestions while the client's back is turned. In that way clients don't have to respond to the suggestions; they can take up the ones they find helpful and simply let the others go by.

What kinds of issues do doctors bring to coaching?

Clinical supervision and coaching are obviously not mutually exclusive and below are some of the problems doctors have presented to me as a coach.

Problems and challenges commonly brought to coaching

- Problems with colleagues (extremely common).
- Stress (due to work overload, conflict, fear of making mistakes).
- Difficulties in getting things done (also common).
- Failing in the job (including disciplinary action/complaints/non-progression in training grades, failing exams).
- Career crises (career decisions, not liking chosen career path, thinking about leaving medicine, adverse events, redundancy or sacking, ill health).
- Applying for new jobs (choosing jobs, CVs, interview skills).
- Difficulties in transition from junior to consultant/GP partner.
- Personal problems that are affecting work.
- Bullying (both targets and perpetrators).

Coaching for learning coaching skills

An inevitable part of coaching, whether in groups or individually, is that you start to learn coaching skills yourself – both how to apply them to your own problems and to those of people you supervise or support. Something that I will often do in group coaching, to help build those skills, is to allow suggestions and advice during question time just so that participants can experience and observe how unhelpful it is. People also learn how to ask questions that help the client, rather than ones which simply increase their own understanding of the situation. As we all know, open questions are much more effective at this than those which require a yes or no answer. Questions beginning with 'how' or 'what' or 'who' are the best. If you take the scenario described above, a better question than 'Why don't you speak to your consultant?' would be, 'Who could you talk to at work about this?' or, 'What are your options in terms of getting support?' If your friend stops to think then you know you've asked a good question. If he answers immediately, he is simply telling you things he already knows, so the question is not helping him.

In development sets, where small groups of professionals get together to tackle individual, often managerial, challenges, I will often ask both clients and other members to assess on a scale of 1–100 how open the questions were, how helpful they were to the clients and the extent to which the clients felt that they had gained what they wanted from the session. When you start to relate the coaching techniques to the results in this way the lessons become much more compelling.

In summary

Doctors tend to be a highly motivated and talented group of people, driven to succeed. Although the work they do is inherently challenging, and often stressful, they work in a culture (especially in hospitals) where they must be seen to be tough and always coping, and where personal support is for wimps. As a result they tend to ignore signs of stress or unhappiness and plough on regardless. Some doctors pay the price of this in the form of breakdowns and performance problems, but for many the consequences are hidden. Because they are hidden, they too can be ignored, and can continue to take their toll on a doctor's mental and physical health over many years. Coaching can certainly help someone to resolve problems of chronic stress and unhappiness, but prevention is better than cure. Regular coaching can help to digest experiences and solve problems before they do serious damage, and it helps you to manage yourself and your work better, increase your self-awareness, improve your relationships and generally increase your effectiveness and happiness at work.

References

Carter, A. J. and West, M. A. (1999) Sharing the burden: team work in health care settings, in J. Firth-Cozens and R. Payne (eds) *Stress in Health Professionals: Psychological and Organizational Causes and Interventions*. London: Wiley.

Firth-Cozens, J. (1999) The psychological problems of doctors, in J. Firth-Cozens and R. Payne (eds) *Stress in Health Professionals: Psychological and Organizational Causes and Interventions*. London: Wiley.

Firth-Cozens, J. (2001) Interventions to improve physicians' wellbeing and patient care, *Social Science and Medicine*, 52: 215–22.

Firth-Cozens, J. (2003) Doctors: their wellbeing and stress, *BMJ*: 326, 670–1.

Jones, J. W., Barge, B. N., Steffy, B. D. *et al.* (1988) Stress and medical malpractice: organizational risk assessment and intervention, *Journal of Applied Psychology*, 4: 727–35.

Myers, I. B. and McCaulley, M. (1985) *Myers-Briggs Type Indicator: A Guide to the Development and Use of the Myers-Briggs Type Indicator*. Palo Alto, CA: Consulting Psychologists Press.

Quine, L. (2002) Workplace bullying in junior doctors: questionnaire survey, *BMJ*, 324: 878–9.

Wall, T. D., Bolden, R. I., Borrill, C. S. *et al.* (1997) Minor psychiatric disorders in NHS trust staff: occupational and gender differences, *British Journal of Psychiatry*, 171: 519–23.

Weinger, M. B. and Ebden, P. (2002) Sleep deprivation and clinical performance, *Journal of the American Medical Association*, 287: 955–8.

9 Supervision skills to enhance appraisal

Sue Morrison and Helen Halpern

Editors' introduction

This chapter explores how clinical supervision can be incorporated into appraisal and be embedded as part of an established and regular review process. While there are many different settings and structures for supervision, we recognize the value of trying to incorporate what it can offer within other pathways of professional development. Integrating different learning and development tools is often synergistic. For example, appraisal often carries the fear of judgement and this fear will block the learning potential inherent in appraisal; a supervisory framework will allow such fears to be articulated and addressed. The writers share both their experience and the ideas about how a supervisory approach based on a collaborative conversation, described more in Chapter 4, can be used in appraisal. It reminds us of the importance of addressing in the agreement between supervisee and supervisor (and appraisee and appraiser) issues related to governance including the very real relationship between what individuals feel able to disclose and how safe they feel (this is developed further in Chapter 12), the need to be self-protective and yet open to the patient's and one's own vulnerability. This chapter offers useful ideas on how supervisory techniques can be used to balance and develop the many differing agendas that are part of appraisal. The overall aim of the chapter is to stimulate the learning and professional development in appraisal to enable what the authors describe as deep learning.

Overview of chapter

We believe that the opportunity for a one-to-one conversation with a colleague during appraisal is a unique chance for some doctors to receive supervision. As appraisal becomes more regulated we describe how it could still afford the possibility for doctors to have a developmental conversation, to reflect on their practice and to present issues for supervision that they may not yet have had the chance to discuss. We hope that appraisers will embrace the more sophisticated approach needed to allow the benefits of appraisal used in this way.

Introduction

Appraisal is a method of evaluating professional behaviour in the workplace, normally including both quantitative and qualitative aspects of performance. It provides an opportunity for a conversation about career focus and progression leading to a personal development plan for professional objectives for the following year (Hands and Hughes 2003). A great deal of attention has been paid to the structural development of NHS appraisal, for example the Revalidation Support Team pilot and related appraiser training (NHS Clinical Governance Support Team Expert Group 2007), but less to the appraisal process and in particular to the conversational skills involved. This can result in a rather dry summative process that is unrewarding for both appraiser and appraisee. We believe that this can be mitigated by including a supervision approach within the appraisal process. Launer (2003a) describes performance appraisal as 'a conversation about how to manage one's learning needs and the wider context of one's career'. His supervision model, Conversations Inviting Change (Launer 2003a), as described in Chapters 4 and 6, can be used in appraisal to enable valuable formative professional development as well as supporting the summative requirements of revalidation. Such formative learning opportunities can facilitate significant learning and step-wise professional progression, as Wass and colleagues (2007) observed. This is applicable in undergraduate and postgraduate settings, encouraging a pathway of professional development that can contribute throughout the medical education continuum towards recertification and relicensing.

Most of our experience and examples derive from primary care, but we believe the principles transfer across different medical specialities.

We are both NHS GP appraisers involved in the training of appraisers and supervisors in the London area. We have found that a structured supervisory conversation with a peer or colleague in an appraisal can enhance its potential as a professional development opportunity for doctors by:

- sharing the locus of control between the appraiser and appraisee;
- restoring a developmental agenda within a regulatory framework that risks becoming focused on superficial targets and competencies;
- helping an appraisee to reflect on his or her professional experience to stimulate the potential for deeper learning;
- encouraging reflection on the complex reality of doctors' working lives.

We use a narrative-based technique that can be applied in a number of situations to develop reflective practice and improve patient care. We describe a 'toolkit' for appraisers wanting to try these supervision techniques.

This type of approach is already happening in some appraisals where appraisee development is prioritized: this may be tacit or conscious, as in a Balint approach (see

Chapter 3) that focuses on the doctor's feelings. However, Launer (2003b) reminds us that many doctors, particularly those in non-training grades, do not have the routine opportunity or expectation of supervision of their practice. We believe that explicitly including supervision as an aspect of appraisal can be particularly useful.

Any approach to formal appraisal will need to map onto the emerging regulatory framework for revalidation and appraisal in the NHS. It is likely that UK doctors will need to demonstrate their continued fitness to practise through the National Revalidation Agenda (Donaldson 2008). A key element of this process will be an annual peer appraisal throughout a five-year cycle. The Revalidation Support Team (Judkins 2010) believes that to be of meaningful quality, appraisers will need to make robust assessments. Generic standards listed in the UK General Medical Council's guide to good medical practice (2006) include skills in appraising and assessing. A variety of approaches are used in other parts of Europe, Australasia and North America, all leading to relicensing and recertification (Merkur *et al.* 2008).

History and background

Although informal supervision has been around for many years, for example in Balint groups, formal approaches only came to prominence in the UK in the last ten years with the introduction of clinical supervision of doctors in training grades. Ideas about appraisal and revalidation that were already infiltrating medicine from the management culture were driven ahead by high-profile reports such as the Bristol Royal Infirmary Inquiry (Kennedy 2001) and Shipman Inquiry (Smith 2002) that demanded regular review of a doctor's fitness to practise.

The political 'new managerialism' of the 1990s brought regulation of the NHS, and a balance between minimum standards and quality practice was sought. The formal need to monitor competencies and politically defined targets tended to follow a 'tick box' culture and the more developmental approaches suffered.

Despite this competency-based climate, some narrative approaches (discussed by Greenhalgh and Hurwitz in 1999) had emerged in medicine in the 1980s with the recognition that human beings tell stories to each other to make sense of their experience and to generate understanding through dialogue. Appraisal of NHS consultants began in 2001, followed by GP appraisals in 2003. The NHS Clinical Governance Support Team Expert Group (2007) was aware of potential limitations:

> If done properly, the process should enhance personal development and learning, but links with revalidation have led to fears about it being used only for assessment.

Roger Neighbour's notion of housekeeping, originally described in *The Inner Consultation* (1987: 235), introduced a framework and prompt for GPs to reflect on their practice, echoing Donald Schön's earlier encouragement in *The Reflective Practitioner* (1983) to reflect on-action and in-action.

While the structures of formal appraisal have sometimes included these informal strands, the focus has remained summative and the locus of control retained by the appraiser. Carl Rogers (Rogers and Freiberg 1994), talking about the locus of control, expresses concern about it being located outside the individual professional: 'knowledge about self is the greatest power ... Fully functioning professionals need a degree of independence to grow'.

Before appraisal started to be used to monitor performance, there was an opportunity for appraisees to get support and guidance from their informal appraiser, to feel helped rather than judged, whereas now they may feel more judged than helped, as Redfern points out (cited in Connor and Pokora 2007: 227): 'They [appraisers] needed the ability to separate these [summative issues] out from the things that the client wanted to work on personally.'

We explore later how the responsibility for managing both the formative and summative agendas may be shared between the appraiser and appraisee.

Supervision in appraisal

The method of supervision we describe (see Chapter 4) helps focus on the complexities and uncertainties of clinical practice, complementing the more usual assessment of unidimensional competencies.

> Many of the parameters we are familiar with are led by processes that can be measured and turned into accessible statistics. This does not always facilitate good general practice, much of which is immeasurable.
>
> (de Kare-Silver 2010)

We believe that a conversational type of appraisal can allow a more sophisticated judgement to contribute to both a formative and summative assessment. However, appraiser and appraisee need to agree what is shared in confidence and what requires disclosure. This situation closely parallels the consultation when the doctor follows strict codes of confidentiality but has a duty to disclose information that is believed to put either the patient or others at significant risk.

CASE EXAMPLE: ANN

Ann, a hospital doctor, shared concerns about one of her senior colleagues in her annual appraisal. She was worried that he was not completing notes adequately and she had concern about some of his clinical skills. She raised this problem in her appraisal and her appraiser asked questions that helped her explore what was bothering her most about this issue and what she might be able to do about it. She discovered that she felt anxious about approaching her colleague, but at the same time aware of her responsibility to protect patient safety. The conversation enabled her to plan to meet her colleague in a way that was not too confrontational. At the end of her appraisal, Ann also considered her options if her colleague was unwilling to discuss this issue. Her appraiser encouraged her to think about a confidential talk with the director of the unit and maybe one of the medical defence unions.

A recent leader in the *BMJ* (Simpson 2011) observes that we are working in an environment where there will be an increasing need '... to create a culture in which clinicians and managers throughout the organisation, at every level, together lead complex patient-centred services' and where 'being able to demonstrate competencies alone will not improve the efficiency and effectiveness of leaders'.

Some doctors say that appraisal as it stands today is good enough to demonstrate a minimum standard of patient care. But others are dissatisfied with the appraisal process, feeling it does not adequately reflect the complexity of doctors' real working lives. Professionalism as defined by the National Clinical Assessment Service (NCAS 2009), 'adherence to an agreed and communicated set of standards', is high on the policy agenda. Competent professionals have to manage issues generated in the arenas of professional practice, individual development and organizational context and also have to maintain the balance between development and governance. We return to this theme later in the chapter. Supervision can be a tool in appraisal for managing these boundaries and issues that sometimes overlap or conflict when seen from different perspectives or in different contexts (see Figure 9.1). The supervision of boundary issues is shared by many other health and social care professions such as social work, psychotherapy and nursing.

From our conversations, we think that many doctors are feeling deprofessionalized by a non-clinical top-down managerial agenda focused on superficial targets and competencies.

Other opportunities for more formative types of appraisal do already exist, notably in GP appraisal as described by Field and Rughani for the RCGP (2008) and Rhydderch and colleagues (2008) and in those using multisource feedback (King 2002) but are

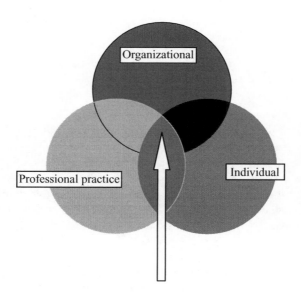

Figure 9.1 The role of supervision

not universal in medical settings. Redfern, as before, describes the use of mentoring techniques in hospital consultant appraisal:

> How was the organisation going to introduce appraisal for all and make it a genuinely valuable exercise rather than just a 'tick box'? The mentors decided to offer to be appraisers ... Peers needed the skills for a confidential conversation.
>
> (Redfern, cited in Connor and Pokora 2007: 227)

There is no convincing direct evidence yet that appraisal improves patient outcomes. However, Chambers and colleagues (2004) are among those who believe systemic changes, brought about by more sophisticated approaches to appraisal such as the encouragement of a culture of reflexivity, outweigh the absence of measurable achievements. This may indirectly improve patient care. The use of supervisory techniques in appraisal helps appraisees understand how their professional development can take place through spending time thinking through work-related issues in more depth.

CASE EXAMPLE: LISA

In her appraisal Lisa brought up the issue of how she worked with colleagues. In particular she was concerned about how to approach team meetings where two colleagues frequently argued with each other about how to manage the care of patients. She felt very uncomfortable in this situation and wanted some ideas about what she could do. Sarah, her appraiser, asked open questions such as:

'What do you think might have made you feel uncomfortable?'
'What do you think your colleagues might say about the situation?'
'What do you imagine other colleagues might do?'
'What have you learned from your responses in similar situations?'

These questions helped Lisa to consider some of the possible factors that might have contributed to the opposing positions held by her colleagues and how these might have been influenced by their differences in gender, age and country of medical training. Lisa was invited to make links with her own experience of being a witness to arguments in other contexts but she felt this was too personal and so it was not pursued in the supervision. Having understood something of her own response to the situation, Lisa felt more able to take a step back when her colleagues argued and to evaluate their comments more objectively.

We suggest that using the framework of Conversations Inviting Change in appraisal can stimulate professional development, maximizing the understandings generated alongside the summative professional judgements. Being able to conceptualize appraisal as a developmental opportunity as well as a necessary bureaucratic activity enhances the potential for effective learning. This in turn may improve the quality of clinical practice. Supervision within appraisal could become a familiar practice, although it requires vigilance to preserve the formative elements of an appraisal that has an assessment function. We believe that Continuing Professional Development (CPD) should be a regular practice throughout professional life, where the techniques of reviewing, monitoring and being supervised become familiar and so embedded in lifelong learning.

Professional development often incorporates new learning. Learning can be classified into three categories:

1   minimum *surface* learning;
2   task-oriented *strategic* learning;
3   significant new understanding through *deep* learning.

Supervision can contribute to learning in each category but becomes a more important tool as learning deepens.

A questioning approach in supervision and appraisal encourages supervisees and appraisees to reflect and probe their professional experience to stimulate the potential for deeper learning (see Figure 9.2)

There is likely to be a tension between formative and summative elements in appraisal and the relationship is not linear. It is possible to use a 'formative conversation' to make a 'summative' assessment, rather than using a competency framework. For example, NHS Quality Improvement Scotland, in reflecting on the quality of their GP appraisal outcomes (2009), found that formative appraisee-centred questions can flush out previously undisclosed or unacknowledged areas of difficulty or excellence. Although a summative judgement has to be made in appraisal, ultimately this type of conversation is more likely to encourage honesty and this may contribute to safer practice and risk avoidance, as illustrated by the following case example.

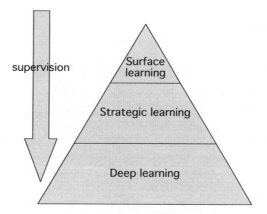

Figure 9.2 Supervision as a facilitator of learning

CASE EXAMPLE: NAT

Nat, a junior partner in a GP practice, was encouraged to set the agenda in his appraisal. His appraiser assured him that they would set aside enough time to cover the necessary summative elements and asked Nat what else he would like to talk about that could make the appraisal meeting useful to him. Nat disclosed some serious concerns about his senior partner's professional behaviour. Afterwards he said that the format, giving him control of pace and content that was comfortable to him, had enabled him to disclose something difficult without feeling he was being interrogated about a potentially inflammatory issue. He said that the conversation had helped move him on from the worry of carrying a problem to formulating possible courses of action for dealing with it.

This approach to appraisal can work well with appraisees who make use of the opportunity to have some supervision about an issue that is troubling them. However, no system can ensure the disclosure of things an appraisee wishes to hide.

The entire appraisal process from preparation to post-appraisal can be an effective piece of supervision leading to change and improved practice. It may also be a focus for collating previous episodes of supervision. The formal conversation may finish at the end of the appraisal meeting, but the thoughts can continue to develop after the event. Some of these may not be shared with the appraiser but continue to resonate with the appraisee, possibly being recorded as significant events or included as narrative in a portfolio.

Our experience is that reflective questioning in a conversationally based appraisal strikes a balance between challenge and an 'appreciative' enquiry (Webb *et al*. 2005) (see Chapter 4) and is more likely to stimulate change and professional development than a purely competency-based assessment. In a narrative-based supervision model, the appraiser manages the process but the content is predominantly driven by the appraisee. It therefore encourages engagement in the more vulnerable or reticent appraisee who is less likely to volunteer information, especially about sensitive issues.

CASE EXAMPLE: KATY

Katy, a GP, returns to work after a year's maternity leave. She is finding it hard to keep up and is tired and forgetful. Katy is anxious about her appraisal with a colleague whom she respects, but fears may judge her poorly. The appraiser begins the appraisal by asking Katy what she would like to get out of their meeting, other than having a 'satisfactory' appraisal. Katy feels the ball to be in her court and can begin to slowly share her concerns in a way that feels safe. She is able to guide the pace of challenge as the appraiser mostly asks her questions that follow on from Katy's own previous statements. This avoids her feeling threatened or overwhelmed, so that she is able to share her lack of confidence and concerns about how to keep up to date and manage her time with her appraiser. Katy and the appraiser consider together the appropriate steps to be included in her professional development plan (PDP).

This example also illustrates the clear distinction that has to be made between performance management and professional development in appraisal: they often overlap in practice. The appraiser needs skills to help the appraisee develop awareness of his or her fullest professional potential, while at the same time keeping an eye open for governance issues: is the doctor's performance safe and fit for practice?

Supervisory techniques can be one way of drawing out these different strands. For example, in appraisal cases that give rise to concern about performance, subsequent data gathering can be orientated towards identifying problems, tracing sources of difficulty and illuminating courses for change. Because appraisal is currently conceived as a peer process its usefulness may be limited if there is defensive behaviour in either the appraiser or appraisee with unwillingness to look at difficulties. Supervision can be a way of challenging patterns of behaviour while continuing to offer support.

Similarly, supervision in appraisal can help an appraisee make changes through offering an opportunity for thinking about and reflecting on options for change. This is facilitated by the appraiser adopting a neutral rather than a judgemental position. Neutrality (Cecchin 1987) is an attitude of mind that promotes curiosity in the appraisal conversation even if the appraiser does not necessarily agree with the position taken by the appraisee on a particular issue. This can be very helpful in preventing the appraiser jumping to premature conclusions about what may be an appropriate course of action for the appraisee to take.

What type of supervision in appraisal?

Chapter 1 describes three main focuses in supervision: educational, supportive and managerial. The conversational techniques we describe are mainly driven by the appraisee's contribution and are most suited to supportive and educational issues. Managerial functions, especially concerning issues of patient safety, technical skill and probity, may be addressed, but sometimes require a more directive approach.

Supervision within appraisal can provide a reflective space to encourage awareness and opportunity for professional development and allow appraisees to monitor themselves. This goes some way to restoring the locus of control to the appraisee, and as Boud (1995: 43) reminds us, '[the] defining feature of self-assessment is that the individual learner ultimately makes a judgement about what has been learned, not that others have no input into it'.

Although appraisal was conceived as a performance management tool, appraisal discussions include a focus on behaviour and attitudes. It provides an opportunity to identify, reorganize and problem solve in relation to clinical cases, working contexts and career progression, and often a combination of all three. Cole (2002: 156–7), working in hospital psychiatry, promotes a solution-based approach:

> [the] positive aim of helping a doctor to develop and progress ... [using] 'solution focussed techniques' and a 'move away from a situation of seeming to question our colleagues' abilities into an exploration of their strengths and skills'.

While it is ideal to keep performance issues (Is this doctor fit to practise?) and development issues (How might this doctor enhance her skills and knowledge?) separate, these are often blurred in real life, so supervisors need to be very clear about maintaining this boundary both for themselves and the supervisee. This may require actively naming this separation of activities within the appraisal. As an appraisee's story unfolds, this approach can help to reconstruct the narrative in a way that may be the key to resolving a particular problem.

CASE EXAMPLE: TIM

Tim, a newly appointed consultant, expressed difficulty and frustration in his relationship with a senior consultant in the unit. He complained that this colleague was remote and aloof and this made Tim feel unable to fully contribute his new ideas and thinking to the unit. After some conversation, it became clear that Tim also tended to work on his own and was seen by others as being rather aloof. Tim came up with the idea of making an effort to be more of a team player, starting by setting up coffee with his senior colleague.

NHS appraisal now reaches most doctors and its structures and processes are continually being refined (Shelly and Judkins 2009). Appraisal for development is part of a broader remit to improve clinical care through the professional development of clinicians. All NHS trusts have a responsibility for the overall quality assurance of appraisal that should underpin good patient care through good staff development (NHS Quality Improvement Scotland 2009).

Three things an appraiser might try to increase the supervision element in future appraisals are:

1   mainly ask questions;
2   keep to the appraisee's story;
3   save any advice to the end of the conversation.

Halpern and McKimm (accessed 2010) have pointed out that there are implicit power differentials between supervisor and supervisee and appraiser and appraisee even in peer arrangements and there needs to be an awareness of how these may impact on the process. Both parties can become disabled by feeling unduly challenged by the other, for example by status, knowledge, seniority, appearance. This could arise if a newly appointed appraiser is assigned a senior, prominent colleague to appraise. In fact, the dynamic may be convoluted with both feeling vulnerable in this situation, the appraiser feeling relatively junior and unskilled and the appraisee maintaining a veneer of authority and arrogance to mask increasing fear of falling out of touch with new changes and developments. By using the technique we describe, these challenging dynamics can be addressed through an initial conversation between appraiser and appraisee to raise awareness of these issues and consider how they may impact on the appraisal process.

Summary

We believe that a narrative-based approach inviting change is a useful way of enhancing NHS appraisal. The method can be integrated relatively simply into the appraisal process and has wide application without major financial implications. It increases the possibility for appraisee-driven professional development as a formative component of appraisal. This is achieved by allowing the appraisee to formulate a new way ahead through dialogue with a colleague who takes a neutral stance. The technique is based on interviewing micro-skills and the responsive nature of the questioning ensures an appraisee-centred approach. This method does not exclude the possibility for the appropriate giving of advice or managing matters of clinical governance.

Narrative-based skills can be applied in a variety of both formal and informal appraisal situations. They have generic applicability and can be used across disciplines and hierarchies. They are not dependent on expertise, status or seniority and can be adapted for use within both short and longer time frames. We believe that this approach to supervision in appraisal is likely to improve job satisfaction and sustainable practice.

References

Boud, D. (1995) *Enhancing Learning through Self Assessment*. Abingdon: Routledge Falmer.

Cecchin, G. (1987) Hypothesizing, circularity and neutrality revisited: an invitation to curiosity, *Family Process*, 26(4): 405–12.

Chambers, R., Tavabie, A., Mohanna, K. and Wakely, G. (2004) *The Good Appraisal Toolkit for Primary Care*. Oxford: Radcliffe.

Cole, M. (2002) Appraising your colleagues, *BMJ Careers*, May: 156–7.

Conlon, M. (2003) Appraisal: the catalyst of personal development, *BMJ*, 327: 389–91.

Connor, M. and Pokora, J. (eds) (2007) *Coaching and Mentoring at Work*. Maidenhead: McGraw-Hill.

De Kare-Silver, N. (2010) *British Journal of General Practice*, DOI: 10.3399/bgjp10X514954.

Donaldson, L. (2008) *Medical Revalidation: Principles and Next Steps*. Available at: HMSO-http://www.dh.gov.uk/en/Publicationsandstatistics/Publications/PublicationsPolicy AndGuidance/DH_086430.

Field, N. and Rughani, A. (2008) *PDP Guidance for Appraisers*. London: Royal College of General Practitioners.

General Medical Council (2006) *Good Medical Practice*, 4th edn. London: GMC.

Greenhalgh, T. and Hurwitz, B. (1999) Why study narrative?, *BMJ*, 318: 48.

Halpern, H. (2009) Supervision and the Johari Window: a framework for asking questions, *Education for Primary Care*, 20(1): 10–14.

Halpern, H. and McKimm, J. (2010) *Supervision E-learning Module*. London Deanery, Faculty Development. Available at: http://faculty.londondeanery.ac.uk/e-learning [accessed 19 September 2010].

Hands, S. and Hughes, M. (2003) A tool to help GP appraisers facilitate educational personal development plans, *Education for Primary Care*, 14: 550–4.

Judkins, K. (2010) *Strengthened Training of Appraisers for Revalidation*. London: NHS Revalidation Support Team. Available at: http://www.revalidationsupport.nhs.uk.

Kennedy, I. (2001) *Learning from Bristol: The Report of the Public Inquiry into Children's Heart Surgery at the Bristol Royal Infirmary 1984–1995*, CM 5207. Available at: http://www.bristol-inquiry.org.uk/ [accessed 26 April 2011].

King, J. (2002) 360 degree appraisal, *BMJ*, 324: S195–6.

Launer, J. (2003a) Practice, supervision, consultancy and appraisal: a continuum of learning, *British Journal of General Practice*, 53(493): 662–6.

Launer, J. (2003b) A narrative-based approach to primary care supervision, in J. Burton and J. Launer (eds) *Supervision and Support in Primary Care*. Oxford: Radcliffe.

Merkur, S., Mladovsky, P., Mossialos, E. and McKee, M. (2008) *Do Lifelong Learning and Revalidation Ensure that Physicians are Fit to Practise?* Geneva: WHO.

NCAS (National Clinical Assessment Service) (2009) *Professionalism: Dilemmas and Lapses*. London: National Patient Safety Agency.

Neighbour, R. (1987) *The Inner Consultation*. Lancaster: MTP Press.

NHS Clinical Governance Support Team Expert Group (2007) *Assuring the Quality of Training for Medical Appraisers*. Available at: http://www.appraisalsupport.nhs.uk.

NHS Quality Improvement Scotland (2009) *Time to Reflect: GP Appraisal in Scotland*. Glasgow/Edinburgh: NHSQIS.

Rhydderch, M., Laugharne, K., Marfell, N. *et al.* (2008) Developing a skills-based model to promote effective appraisal discussions amongst GPs in Wales, *Education for Primary Care*, 19: 496–505.

Rogers, C. and Freiberg, H.J. (1994) *Freedom to Learn*. New Jersey: Prentice Hall.

Schön, D. (1983) *The Reflective Practitioner*. New York: Basic Books.

Shelly, M. and Judkins, K. (2009) *Assuring the Quality of Medical Appraisal for Revalidation*. London: Revalidation Support Team. Available at: http://www.appraisalsupport. nhs.uk/.

Simpson, J. (2011) Editorial, *Clinical Leader*. Available at: http://www.leadership. londondeanery.ac.uk/home/links/downloads/Clinical%20Leader-Darzi%20and%20 Leadership.pdf [accessed 24 May 2012].

Smith, J. (2002) www.dh.gov.uk/Consultations/LiveConsultations/fs/en [accessed 9 September 2010].

Sparrow, N. (2003) *Principles of GP Appraisal*. London: Royal College of General Practitioners.

Wass, V., Bowden, R. and Jackson, N. (2007) The principles of assessment design, in N. Jackson, A. Jamieson and A. Khan (eds) *Assessment in Medical Education and Training: A Practical Guide*. London: Routledge.

Webb, L., Preskill, H. and Coughlan, A. (2005) Bridging two disciplines: applying appreciative inquiry to evaluative practice, *AI Practitioner, The International Journal of Appreciative Inquiry Best Practice*, 1–4: 2–3.

10 Effective supervision: the evidence base

Maggie Stanton and Christine Dunkley

Editors' introduction

When compiling the different chapters, we realized that many contributors had written from their extensive personal experience but that there were few mentions of the evidence that exists. We were keen to give a fuller picture of the benefits of supervision to both doctors and patients, so we asked the authors if they would be willing to fill the gap. Their survey of the literature highlights informative studies while showing how difficult it is to conduct good research on the efficacy of supervision. This is partly because of definitions, partly because of the multiple stakeholders and partly because there are no clear criteria for outcomes and how to measure them. The authors present useful evidence for individuals, teams and organizations that want to explore the benefits of engaging in, or providing supervision. As with so much of medicine, more robust research is desirable and this chapter links the positive experience of supervision, documented throughout this book, to the important research questions those interested in supervision would like addressed.

Overview of chapter

Clinical supervision has become more evident in the medical profession during the last decade. Supervision is now a requirement for all doctors on training grades, but availability and quality remains variable. Provision of supervision is not yet established as routine throughout the medical sector and the evidence base is only now beginning to develop at a faster pace. In this chapter we have reviewed the literature across the helping professions and summarized research that would be of interest to those working in medicine. We have looked at three major issues: what is effective for the supervisee, for the organization and, most importantly, for the patient. Features of effective supervision sessions include a supportive relationship, and a client-focused agenda. We describe how quality of supervision might be measured reliably utilizing validated scales. There is evidence linking good quality supervision to reduced burnout and staff retention, but more research is needed to establish the link between supervision and patient outcomes. Finally we draw on our own reflections as both supervisors and trainers, sharing our observation that willingness of all participants to be emotionally present is the key factor in successful supervision.

Introduction

Supervision is increasingly seen as important in maintaining the well-being of staff and providing quality care to patients. For most professionals in the health and social care sector there will be a requirement from their professional body that they undertake supervision (not just during training but as an ongoing requirement for professional development and continued registration), and the majority would agree that this is a necessary activity. Kilminster and Jolly (2000: 827) point out: 'Clinical supervision has a vital role in post-graduate and, to some extent, undergraduate medical education. However it is probably the least investigated, discussed and developed aspect of clinical education.'

Researchers have been seeking to corroborate the usefulness of supervision through scientific enquiry, to answer questions such as:

- What exactly is supervision?
- What are the challenges of developing an evidence base?
- What is the uptake of supervision and what gets in the way?
- What are the effects of supervision on the supervisee?
- What constitutes effective supervision?
- Is a supervised professional more likely to achieve better outcomes with patients?

When looking at the evidence base it is helpful to consider studies from across the healthcare professions as they offer insights into what the important issues and approaches are. Research in this area has proved challenging, with the evidence base for the efficacy of supervision traditionally being heavy on opinion and light on evidence (Kavanagh *et al.* 2002). At the end of the chapter we include a section informed by our personal experience from our own practice, as this addresses areas that we believe are important for further research.

What is supervision?

Full descriptions of supervision have already been addressed in other chapters of this book (see Chapter 1). Arriving at a universally agreed definition that can be used in research has been problematic. There is considerable overlap between clinical supervision and teaching, coaching, mentoring or training. Researchers have reviewed studies to try and standardize definitions without success. There is a common theme across disciplines, however, of definitions that include the 'formative, normative and restorative' functions of supervision, which can be loosely translated as education, administration and support (Milne 2007). In addition, definitions used in medical studies often include an emphasis on maximizing patient safety (Kilminster and Jolly 2000). Milne points out in his book *Evidence-Based Clinical Supervision* (2009) that we need a shared understanding of what supervision is and is not. He argues that, unless we have a definition that is specific, can be operationalized and measured, we will not be able to carry out robust research in this area.

Challenges for developing the evidence base

There are potentially five parties involved in the supervisory relationship: the supervisee, the supervisor, the patients, the employer and the professional organization or registering body (Kavanagh *et al.* 2002). All may have competing expectations and demands. Without clarity on rationale, objectives and components of supervision it is difficult to identify outcomes, and therefore to devise appropriate measures.

Gilmore (1999) carried out a review of studies on the effectiveness of clinical supervision in the UK and found the majority were evaluations on the process, rather than outcome of supervision. Satisfaction surveys rated by supervisees or supervisors are often used to assess effectiveness of supervision rather than direct observation of participants, or measurement of clinical improvements for patients (Gonsalvez *et al.* 2002).

Studies are often of poor quality, with methodological problems ranging from the lack of validated measures, through small sample size, to the use of repeated tests of statistical significance without the necessary adjustment to the significance levels. Also studies of practitioners in training are more plentiful than studies of experienced practitioners, which could skew findings (Schoenwald *et al.* 2009).

An important step in improving the quality of research in this area has been the development of validated measures such as the Manchester Clinical Supervision Scale (MCSS) (Winstanley 2000). This has seven empirically derived domains that evaluate supervision in terms of:

- trust/rapport;
- supervisor advice/support;
- improved care/skills;
- importance/value of supervision;
- finding time;
- personal issues;
- reflection.

Thirty six items are rated from strongly disagree to strongly agree, giving a total score. It is the most common measure of effectiveness used in recent studies. While it has improved research in this area it still relies on self-report with all the limitations that brings.

Gonge and Buus (2011) not only emphasize the methodological limitations of research but also highlight the lack of theoretical orientation. They have proposed a model for analysing and understanding the possible benefits of supervision. The pathway they outline suggests participation in supervision will impact on perceived effectiveness of supervision (for the supervisee), which in turn will impact on the benefits of clinical supervision (for the patient). The study they carried out to investigate this model provided some evidence for the pathway, but it was not possible to determine the direction of travel as, for example, positive ratings for effective supervision may be a consequence of frequent participation but it could equally be that positive ratings of effectiveness motivate frequent attendance.

Uptake of supervision

Factors affecting uptake

- Supervision not available
- Lack of protected time
- Competing demands
- Suspicion
- Viewed as being for lower grades only
- Travel distance

In medicine, as with other professions, there is wide variability in the availability and uptake of supervision (Grant *et al.* 2003; Orman and Thornton 2010). Evidence for participation in supervision is surprisingly scarce. Buus and Gonge (2009) carried out a review of studies of participation in supervision by psychiatric nurses and found it ranged from 33 per cent to 81 per cent (median 73 per cent). Given that not everyone will return their questionnaire, the actual rates of participation are probably lower. They point out that the view of supervision in the literature is that it is generally seen as a 'good thing' but studies reported mixed views from nurses.

In a study by Buus *et al.* (2011) nurses reported supervision helped them to gain a new perspective on a problem when a case was not moving forward. This provided emotional support and increased energy to work on the problem. Despite this they said it did not have much impact on their practice because they found it hard to take time to attend due to the demands of their work. They emphasized the need for management to prioritize and protect time for supervision.

Lack of time can be one of the many barriers to the uptake of supervision. There is variability in how much time is given to supervision, that with some surveys showing their 25–30 per cent of mental health professionals receive no supervision and, when supervision is available, sessions are often short and infrequent. Typically more experienced staff members receive less supervision. Competing work demands, travel distances and lack of appropriate supervisors are all given as reasons for problems in accessing supervision. Other barriers include lack of organizational structure or policies to support supervision (Bush 2005) or misconceptions, such as that it would only apply to junior staff (Carney 2005). Kilminster and Jolly (2000) highlight that the boundaries between management supervision and clinical supervision can be blurred, which may account for why supervision is not always met with a positive response, with some staff reporting being suspicious about how supervision will be used (Lyth 2000).

Benefits of supervision for supervisees

A number of studies have looked at the outcome of supervision in terms of positive impact for the supervisee. Wheeler and Richards (2007) have produced a systematic review of studies relating to psychotherapy supervision, showing a range of benefits. Common themes were that supervision improved supervisees' self-confidence, awareness and skill.

Satisfaction with supervision has been linked to reduced rates of burnout (see Chapter 7). In one study Edwards *et al.* (2006) conducted a survey of 817 community mental health nurses in Wales. Participants completed the Maslach Burnout Inventory (Maslach and Jackson 1986) and the Manchester Clinical Supervision Scale. There was a significant negative correlation between scores on the MCSS and both emotional exhaustion and depersonalization scales on the Maslach Burnout Inventory.

Another widely reported finding is the relationship between supervision and job satisfaction. In a questionnaire survey of 136 participants Gonge and Buus (2011) found perceived effectiveness of supervision was associated with increased job satisfaction, vitality and rational coping. It is important to note that it is the perceived effectiveness and not supervision *per se* that produced this result, as this highlights the importance not just of providing supervision but of supervision being seen as effective.

What makes supervision effective?

Most of the research relies on preference ratings rather than direct observation and observed outcomes. What seems to be effective in the content of supervision largely depends on whichever function takes priority. If the function is to enhance clinical skill in delivering an evidence-based intervention then feedback and direction are most likely to be effective. This is most likely to be achieved through utilizing techniques such as direct observation, reviewing video or audio recordings. Research has shown that professionals often prefer this kind of supervision early in their career, but as time goes on they value more relational activities, with support and validation (Guest and Beutler 1988).

Kavanagh *et al.* (2002) also found that what supervisees want from supervision changes with their level of experience and type of case seen. Less experienced supervisees preferred directive or skills-focused supervision. Experienced therapists also liked this type of supervision when struggling with a difficult clinical issue, but generally preferred reflecting on issues raised in therapy.

Edwards *et al.* (2005) found supervision was evaluated more positively where sessions lasted over an hour and took place at least monthly. The quality of supervision was also perceived as higher where nurses had chosen their supervisor and where sessions took place away from the workplace.

Accurso *et al.* (2011) collected data from routine supervision sessions in community-based child mental health. Both supervisee and supervisor submitted their analysis of the session content. There was rough agreement between supervisors and supervisees that across 130 supervision sessions the content was:

- 25 per cent therapy interventions and approaches;
- 25 per cent case formulation;
- 11 per cent client alliance;
- 11 per cent administration;
- 11 per cent case-management issues;
- 6 per cent supervisee professional roles;
- 5 per cent crisis assessment;
- 4 per cent supervisory relationship.

Both supervisees and supervisors assessed that in many sessions no evidence-based content was discussed at all. There was agreement that too little time was spent discussing client alliance and interventions.

Within the nursing profession there has been a huge movement towards reflective practice (Kinsella 2009) which guides the focus of the session around a set of self-reflective questions. The anecdotal evidence that these groups are helpful is abundant, but currently without any firm evidence base. A study of psychology trainees in reflective practice groups showed that while the majority of participants found them helpful for their professional development, others reported finding the group distressing. The authors concluded that smaller group sizes and more skilled facilitation were advisable to minimize the likelihood of distress (Knight *et al.* 2010). Balint groups also emphasize the importance of skilled leaders for their groups (see Chapter 3).

Example of reflective practice supervision in a multidisciplinary group

In this case the members of the supervision group belong to a multidisciplinary team from a drug and alcohol charity. The team runs groups and provides individual caseworkers. The supervisor is a health professional from outside the charity. Groups are monthly with caseworkers and group leaders.

Supervisees are invited to bring some aspect of their casework to form the subject of their reflective practice. This is usually an incident around which they noticed some discrepancy between the desired outcome and what took place. They write this on a supervision form which they keep with them during the session. The agenda is set at the start of the session around the number of incidents and any similarities between them. Sometimes more than one worker is having a problem with the same case.

The supervisor guides the discussion around the following questions: What happened? What did you notice, internally and externally? What did you do?

What are your reflections now? What would you do differently if this happened again? The focus is on self-reflection utilizing the group to explore feelings, relationships and values in order to identify options. The supervisees are encouraged to develop a sense of their own 'internal supervisor'. Contributions of other group members allow different perspectives on each issue. There is no expectation that the supervisor is an expert in the field.

At the end of the session participants complete the remainder of their supervision form asking if they got the help they needed, and asking them to state ways in which their practice might change in response to the session. These forms are copied for the supervisor and then group members retain the originals for future reference. In this way both supervisees and supervisor can see if patterns recur over time.

The presence of a supervisor who holds no managerial responsibility is important.

(Cutliffe and Hyrkas 2006)

Sloan (2005) reviewed the literature and found that characteristics that supervisors see as important to supervision are:

- making specific suggestions about interventions;
- giving feedback on performance;
- providing a non-judgemental environment;
- promoting autonomy;
- listening;
- being committed to supervision.

Detailed feedback was found to be effective in study by Beck (1986). In this study an intensive training programme was followed by clinical practice. Those with supervision maintained their skills, while those without supervision returned to pre-course levels within nine months. Gist (1987) showed supervisees audio or visual recordings of their own sessions with clients. The supervisees found this more effective than feedback alone. Ways of giving feedback in different settings and with limited time is discussed in Chapter 5. Giving and receiving feedback was also seen as important in a study by Bogo *et al.* (2011). They held focus groups for seventy six staff from different professional backgrounds to assess the impact of supervision during a period of organizational change. Participants agreed that it was important supervision was regular and that those who provided it were able to teach new treatment skills and had expert knowledge about interventions for the specific client group. They found it helpful to discuss their feelings and struggles and to gain a sense of perspective on their competence when they were lacking in confidence.

Goals should be:

- specific;
- attainable;
- measurable.

Feedback should be:

- timely;
- clear;
- balanced between positive and negative.

Kilminster *et al.* (2007), in their guidance for effective supervision in the medical profession, point to helpful supervisory behaviours such as:

- giving direct guidance
- joint problem solving
- offering feedback
- linking theory to practice
- providing support
- having a supervision contract

They hypothesize that the supervision relationship is probably the single most important factor for effective supervision (Kilminster and Jolly 2000).

There is much emphasis in the literature on the importance of goal setting and using goals to structure feedback. Auty (2005) highlighted the benefits of setting clear achievable tasks when supervising in general practice. Lehrman-Waterman and Ladany (2001) report that effective goal setting and feedback was associated with a stronger working alliance, enhanced self-efficacy and increased supervisee satisfaction with supervision. Gonsalvez *et al.* (2002) suggest there should be specific objectives around knowledge, skill, attitude and relationship factors and that these will then determine the content, resources, methods, assessment and evaluation criteria needed. They suggest this approach can be used at the macro level to plan supervision programmes and at the micro level in relation to specific supervisor/supervisee arrangements.

Supervisor training

There is very little in the literature about supervisor training. Kavanagh *et al.* (2003), in a survey of allied mental health practitioners in Queensland, found only 33 per cent of supervisors had received supervisor training and only 18 per cent had received more than twelve hours of training. They carried out a randomized controlled trial to investigate the impact of supervisor training on supervision. Results showed that training supervisees and their supervisors together resulted in more areas being specified in the supervision agreement and a lower frequency of perceived problems as rated by the supervisors. The frequency of use of beneficial strategies dropped over time for all conditions. One possible explanation could be that after training the supervisors did not receive supervision themselves to support implementation.

Supervisors often recognize their own need for training. In a study of attending doctors in university and district teaching hospitals in the Netherlands (Busari and Koot 2007) the doctors felt the overall quality of supervision was satisfactory but rated themselves as requiring training in a number of areas of supervision, e.g. providing feedback.

Evaluation of supervisor training is an area worth focusing on in the future as shown by Hyrkas *et al.* (2006). They carried out a questionnaire survey of healthcare professionals with at least six months' experience of supervision. The response rate was 62 per cent with 799 respondents. Supervisors who had had supervision training were rated significantly more highly on a range of evaluation measures than their non-trained colleagues.

Efficacy for patients

Few studies have looked at the efficacy of supervision in terms of outcomes for the patient despite Ellis and Ladany stating as early as 1997 that this is the 'acid test' of supervision (1997: 485). In their review of the literature, Wheeler and Richards (2007) found that only two of eighteen studies looked at this. In one, no effect was reported and in the other, changes were noted but how far this result was able to be generalized was limited by the single case study design.

There is some evidence that lack of supervision leads to poor outcomes. McKee and Black (1992) found that there were higher death rates associated with lack of supervision for junior doctors in specialities that require more technical skill, such as anaesthetics and trauma work. This would suggest that it is not sufficient to have hours of training without ongoing support and performance feedback.

It seems logical that where a clinical procedure has achieved its own evidence base through randomized controlled trials (RCTs) then one role of supervision would be to ensure that the practitioner adheres to the standard model of care. This type of supervision is well known in treatment trials where it is necessary to ensure that the treatment is delivered to the highest possible standard. In these trials practitioners may be videoed and the tape reviewed to check what is being done. The same level of supervision, however, is often missing in routine care. Experienced practitioners may consider that it is unnecessary, and yet a parallel can be drawn with attaining a driving licence, where over time precision is lost and bad habits can creep in. On the other hand, expertise develops over time and practitioners may feel deskilled with constant adherence monitoring. Somers *et al.* (1994) suggest that in the highly competitive medical profession doctors have to appear competent very quickly, and that this pressure can interfere with openness to corrective feedback.

Harkness and Hensley (1991) showed that the focus of supervision can have a dramatic effect on client satisfaction. They compared mixed focus supervision sessions (no fixed agenda) with supervision sessions guided by a set of client-focused questions such as 'What does the client want? What are you doing to help? Does the client think it is helping?' Clients whose therapists were in receipt of client-focused supervision showed up to 30 per cent improvement in satisfaction ratings. There were limitations to the study such as the small sample size, but these results provide promising indications for the use of protocols within supervision sessions, and especially those related to client outcomes.

Heaven *et al.* (2006) used a randomized controlled trial to see whether supervision had an effect on the implementation of a training course. Sixty one clinical nurse specialists attended training in communication skills for three days. Half were randomly allocated to attend supervision weekly for four weeks (twelve hours total) and half did not. Assessments were carried out before the trial, after the supervision and three months later. Within-group effects showed that only those who attended supervision had evidence of the use of skills taught on the course, with real and simulated patients. Those who attended supervision were found to significantly increase their use of skills taught on the course, i.e. open questions, negotiation and exploration skills, which resulted in them identifying more of their clients' concerns. Those who did not attend supervision had a decline in skills over the same time period. Despite the fact that there were no statistically significant differences between groups, i.e. between those that received supervision and those that did not, the within-group effects indicate that supervision made a real-world difference in the skills of nurses over time. The authors hypothesize that four weeks was too short to show a difference between groups.

Bradshaw *et al.* (2007) found that there were greater increases in positive attitudes by nurses, greater levels of knowledge and greater reduction in symptoms for patients when psychiatric nurses were provided with workplace supervision to implement a psychosocial intervention.

There are indications that research in this area is improving. Schoenwald *et al.* (2009) carried out a prospective, longitudinal study which looked at a number of factors that influenced outcome in a treatment programme for 1888 youths with serious antisocial behaviour. Supervision was provided for 429 therapists by 122 clinical supervisors. They found that greater therapist adherence was predicted by the dimension of supervisor focus on adherence to treatment principles. Changes in youth behaviour were predicted by two supervision dimensions (i.e. adherence to the structure and process of supervision and focus on clinical development).

Personal reflections on supervising in the medical profession

In reviewing the literature it is also helpful to review our own overwhelmingly positive experiences of both training and supervising with colleagues in the medical profession. We realize this personal evidence is at one end of the spectrum of the robustness of evidence, but like clinical experience it is important it is not lost, both for its own value and to inform how more rigorous studies can be conducted. Successful supervision requires supervisor and supervisee to be present, both physically and emotionally. Physical presence can be difficult enough – time pressures in the NHS are huge. The emphasis is often on meeting targets, increasing throughput and decreasing waiting times. To take time out for reflection can seem at best a luxury and at worst a waste of time. And yet those clinicians who do manage to make time report a sense that something has been gained – though that 'added value' can be hard to capture in a scientific study.

Feedback we have received shows that clinicians value the following:

- An opportunity to think about improving on what is currently being done. Trainees may have lots of time allocated to this which falls away drastically on qualification. Yet even very experienced clinicians can always identify ways to improve if they have the space and time to apply themselves to this question.

- Taking a different perspective. Supervisees talk of 'stepping back' from the case or situation and looking through fresh eyes. The fact of the supervisor coming from a different discipline can not only provide an alternative viewpoint but also remove hierarchical structures that may inhibit expression of thought or feeling.
- Gaining support and validation. Where the medical profession is used to enquiries into mistakes or failure, it can be less common to review good practice and difficult decisions which did not result in a negative outcome.

For the supervisee to benefit from each of these aspects of supervision we return to the concept of being emotionally present. This requires both supervisee and supervisor to do the following:

- Allow vulnerability – not an easy task in a profession where remaining cool under pressure is positively reinforced. Vulnerability may feel like a weakness.
- Disclose feelings. The clinician is in real relationships with patients and colleagues, but these are often constrained by protocols and hierarchies. Medical professionals can describe a sense of loneliness that comes with responsibility. Natural responses such as worry, dislike, disgust or confusion can be seen in the working environment as unprofessional, yet there is often relief when these feelings can be expressed in a safe supervisory relationship. Peer supervision can be really helpful when both parties are able to match the other's disclosure (see Chapter 6).
- Be open to feedback. In a pressured competitive environment this can feel like criticism and it is the task of both supervisor and supervisee to develop trust so that feedback is a positive experience.

Knowledge of the evidence base assists the supervisor to remain focused on the function of supervision. Supervision does not become 'offloading' because the questions always remain: how can this feeling, response or insight help us to improve our contact or intervention next time? What can we do differently, and how can we monitor the outcome for patients? We strive to balance a human, accepting style with a focus on improvement that can be measured. Keeping this balance ensures that supervision is both well attended and valued.

Conclusion

The evidence base for supervision has grown over the years and there is much to be learned from looking at research across disciplines. In our experience of providing supervision to members of the medical profession it is evident that they are keen to provide high quality interventions that produce good outcomes for their patients. The use of supervision contracts can help with this as it provides a forum to discuss expectations and agree the process and content of supervision. The trend for more robust research needs to continue, despite the many challenges for research in this area, if we are to pass the 'acid test' that Ellis and Ladany (1997) highlighted. The evidence that is currently available shows an advantage to both practitioners and patients when the clinician engages in effective supervision. There is a growing consensus on the factors that promote effectiveness in supervision, but less evidence on the mechanisms by which benefits filter through to patients. The medical profession faces increasing pressure to streamline and improve patient care while retaining staff, so it is important to understand the role that supervision plays in this process. It is vital that further well-designed studies are conducted in order to continue to expand the evidence base, and that practitioners continue to audit the level, quality and outcomes of the supervision that they receive.

References

Accurso, E., Taylor, R. and Garland, A. (2011) Evidence-based practices addressed in community-based children's mental health supervision, *Training and Education in Professional Psychology*, 5(2): 88–96.

Auty, S. (2005) GP practice: supervising staff to everyone's benefit, *GP: General Practitioner*, 4 January, 30–5.

Beck, A. T. (1986) Cognitive therapy: a sign of retrogression or progress, *Behaviour Therapist*, 9: 2–3.

Bogo, M., Paterson, J., Tufford, L. and King, R. (2011) Supporting front-line practitioners' professional development and job satisfaction in mental health and addiction, *Journal of Interprofessional Care*, 25: 209–14.

Bradshaw, T., Butterworth, A. and Mairs, H. (2007) Does structured supervision during psychological intervention education enhance outcome for mental health nurses and the service users they work with?, *Journal of Psychiatric and Mental Health Nursing*, 14: 4–12.

Busari, J. O. and Koot, B. G. (2007) Quality of clinical supervision as perceived by attending doctors in university and district teaching hospitals, *Medical Education*, 41: 957–64.

Bush, T. (2005) Overcoming the barriers to effective supervision, *Nursing Times*, 101(2): 38–41.

Buus, N. and Gonge, H. (2009) Empirical studies of clinical supervision in psychiatric nursing: a systematic literature review and methodological critique, *International Journal of Mental Health Nursing*, 18(4): 250–64.

Buus, N., Angel, S., Traynor, M. and Gonge, H. (2011) Psychiatric nursing staff members' reflections on participating in group-based clinical supervision: a semistructured interview study, *International Journal of Mental Health Nursing*, 20: 95–101.

Carney, S. (2005) Clinical supervision in a challenging behavior unit, *Nursing Times*, 101(47): 32–4.

Cutliffe, J. and Hyrkas, K. (2006) Multidisciplinary attitudinal positions regarding clinical supervision: a cross-sectional study, *Journal of Nursing Management*, 14(8): 617–37.

Edwards, D., Cooper, L., Burnard, P. *et al.* (2005) Factors influencing the effectiveness of supervision, *Journal of Psychiatric and Mental Health Nursing*, 12: 405–14.

Edwards, D., Burnard, P., Hannigan, B. *et al.* (2006) Clinical supervision and burnout: the influence of clinical supervision for community mental health nurses, *Journal of Clinical Nursing*, 15(8): 1007–15.

Ellis, M. V. and Ladany, N. (1997) Inferences concerning supervisees and clients in clinical supervision: an integrative review, in C. E. Watkins (ed.) *Handbook of Psychotherapy Supervision*. New York: Wiley.

Gilmore, A. (1999) *Review of the United Kingdom Evaluative Literature on Clinical Supervision in Nursing and Health Visiting*. London: UKCC.

Gist, A. (1987) Self-efficacy: implications for organizational behaviour and human resource management, *Academic Management Review*, 12: 472–85.

Gonge, H. and Buus, N. (2011) Model for investigating the benefits of clinical supervision in psychiatric nursing, *International Journal of Mental Health Nursing*, 20: 102–11.

Gonsalvez, C. J., Oades, L. G. and Freestone, J. (2002) The objectives approach to clinical supervision: towards integration and empirical evaluation, *Australian Psychologist*, 37(1): 68–77.

Grant, J., Kilminster, S., Jolly, B. and Cottrell, D. (2003) Clinical supervision of SpRs: where does it happen, when does it happen and is it effective?, *Medical Education*, 37: 140–8.

Guest, P. and Beutler, L. (1988) Impact of psychotherapy supervision on therapist orientation and values, *Journal of Consulting and Clinical Psychology*, 56(5): 653–8.

Harkness, D. and Hensley, H. (1991) Changing the focus of social work supervision, *Social Work*, 36: 506–13.

Heaven, C., Clegg, J. and Maguire, P. (2006) Transfer of communication skills training from workshop to workplace: the impact of clinical supervision, *Patient Education and Counseling*, 60: 313–25.

Hyrkas, K., Appelqvist-Schmidlechner, K. and Haataja, R. (2006) Efficacy of clinical supervision: influence on job satisfaction, burnout and quality of care, *Nursing and Healthcare Management and Policy*, 55(4): 521–35.

Kavanagh, D., Spence, S., Wilson, J. and Crow, N. (2002) Achieving effective supervision, *Drug and Alcohol Review*, 21: 247–52.

Kavanagh, D., Spence, S., Strong, J. *et al.* (2003) Supervision practices in allied mental health: a staff survey, *Mental Health Services Research*, 5: 187–95.

Kilminster, S. and Jolly, B. (2000) Effective supervision in clinical practice settings: a literature review, *Medical Education*, 34: 827–40.

Kilminster, S., Cottrell, D., Grant, J. and Jolly, B. (2007) AMEE guide no. 27: effective educational and clinical supervision, *Medical Teacher*, 29: 2–19.

Kinsella, E. (2009) Professional knowledge and epistemology of reflective practice, *Nursing Philosophy*, 11: 395–409.

Knight, K., Sperlinger, D. and Maltby, M. (2010) Exploring the personal and professional impact of reflective practice groups: a survey of 18 cohorts from a UK clinical psychology training course, *Clinical Psychology and Psychotherapy*, 17(5): 427–37.

Lehrman-Waterman, D. and Ladany, N. (2001) Development and validation of the evaluation process within supervision inventory, *Journal of Counseling Psychology*, 48(2): 168–77.

Lyth, G. M. (2000) Clinical supervision: a concept analysis, *Journal of Advanced Nursing*, 31: 722–9.

McKee, M. and Black, N. (1992) Does the current use of junior doctors in the United Kingdom affect the quality of medical care?, *Social Science Medicine*, 34: 548–58.

Maslach, C. and Jackson, S. (1986) *The Maslach Burnout Inventory*, 2nd edn. Palo Alto, CA: Consulting Psychologists Press.

Milne, D. (2007) An empirical definition of clinical supervision, *British Journal of Clinical Psychology*, 46: 437–47.

Milne, D. (2009) *Evidence-Based Clinical Supervision: Principles and Practice*. Chichester: BPS Blackwell.

Orman, S. A. and Thornton, V. J. (2010) Analysis of junior doctor supervision in Australasian emergency departments, *Emergency Medicine Australasia*, 22: 301–9.

Schoenwald, S. K., Sheidow, A. J. and Chapman, J. E. (2009) Clinical supervision in treatment transport: effects on adherence and outcome, *Journal of Consulting and Clinical Psychology*, 77(3): 410–21.

Sloan, G. (2005) Clinical supervision: beginning the supervisory relationship, *British Journal of Nursing*, 14(17): 918–22.

Somers, P., Muller, J., Saba, G., Draisin, J. and Shore, W. (1994) Reflections on action: medical students' accounts of their implicit beliefs and strategies in the context of one-to-one clinical teaching, *Academic Medicine*, 69: 584–7.

Wheeler, S. and Richards, K. (2007) The impact of clinical supervision on counsellors and therapists, their practice and their clients: a systematic review of the literature, *Counselling and Psychotherapy Research*, 7(1): 54–65.

Winstanley, J. (2000) *Manchester Clinical Supervision Scale User Guide*. Sydney: Osman Consulting Pty Ltd.

11 The supervisee's perspective

Patricia Ridsdale

Editors' introduction

When starting to edit this book we were aware that to make it more than a tool for existing supervisors, it needed to provide sufficient information for doctors thinking of supervision or just looking for support in their work to make a decision whether or not to try it. As such we were mindful of our own early experience of supervision, the excitement, challenges and sense of discovery. We knew we wanted this to be reflected in the book and are pleased that someone, more in touch with their early experience than us, has written this chapter. We reflected on placing it at the beginning of the book but decided that the more personal chapter about the benefits might carry more weight if the differing approaches to supervision were described first. The account mentions many important themes like powerlessness, bereavement and endings, handling uncertainty, not being good enough, which can be very much part of a supervisory dynamic. These are often difficult to talk about and yet this chapter introduces these from a supervisee's perspective. While all that has been written might help a doctor weigh up the benefits of supervision, ultimately the author is encouraging readers to try it and see.

Overview of chapter

My hope for those reading this chapter is that it will go some way to demystifying supervision and, if you are not receiving it already, inspire you to go ahead and try it. My experience is that it has enhanced both my working and home life and has helped me to put the art back into medicine when I was struggling to remember sometimes why I went into medicine in the first place.

Introduction

Many medical colleagues question why I have supervision. Given how much I have come to value supervision and how I consider it an essential part of my working life, I am puzzled and I want to challenge their views. Some ask why I feel I need it, others are sceptical of the time investment and still others express a fear of exposing potential weakness or looking silly. I have found supervision to be a thoroughly positive experience and one that has supported my practice on a daily basis. In this chapter I write from the experience of being a supervisee and I will give some idea of what may happen in supervision and the common themes that I have encountered. By the end I want you to understand why supervision is an essential part of my practice and I want to make a case for supervision being part of all doctors' practice.

I imagine most GPs have had patients who bring problem after problem. No matter how hard we try to help them they just keep returning with something else. We somehow know we are never quite getting to the root of the problem. I liken it to the analogy of the octopus and the string bag – no matter how fast you stuff the octopus into the bag, an arm just keeps popping out.

Until I was offered the opportunity for supervision through my NHS general practice I struggled, like my colleagues, with many octopi. Supervision gave me a chance to step out of the struggle and look at the dynamics of the consultation in a safe and supportive environment. This has enabled me to be more confident in consultations with patients, exploring areas that the patient has brought into the consultation environment which have either passed unnoticed or I have not had the confidence to acknowledge and bring into the discussion. This has facilitated a fuller, more rounded conversation and, I believe, benefited patients in the understanding and interpretation of their problems.

In general practice the opportunity to discuss consultations in detail is less common after our training is completed. There are fewer ways of having support, though in some areas young GPs' groups and non-principals' groups are becoming more popular. My experience is that supervision gives an opportunity to reflect deeply and provides feedback and support, posing questions that may need to be considered to explore the consultation fully.

Initially I felt exposed and vulnerable to criticism and I imagine this has, or could, put some doctors off supervision. However, this feeling actually settled in the first session as I realized just how beneficial to me and my patients this way of working would be. Within the first supervision group we were all bringing very similar problems. These included time management, often running late, dealing with the patient with a list of problems, difficult relationships with colleagues and patients who provoked irritation or frustration or a sense of being stuck and unable to progress.

What is happening in supervision

Good medical practice (General Medical Council 2010) suggests that we should be reviewing significant events both personally and within our working environment.

We may already be doing this on an informal basis when we discuss critical incidents or complaints as a one-off, or more formally seek the advice and support of a colleague or with a nominated supervisor (see Chapter 5).

While I have found one-to-one supervision very focused and productive, I have found that group supervision of regular members develops a character and 'flavour' of its own, which can be both affirming and challenging. It can be quite exciting to taste what is in the mixture in an ongoing group and often recurrent themes will emerge (see Chapter 3). The group itself helps to stimulate awareness of what exactly is taking place, both expressed explicitly and hidden beneath the surface and either unnamed or unacknowledged.

Sometimes, for example, we don't notice the simple things that others may note in the way we present a case or talk about a particular patient or situation, the slight wobble in the voice, the spontaneous denial or faster speech which may indicate something hidden. Having a witness or witnesses to our telling of the consultation can gently explore our way of telling and pick up unrecognized issues reflected in the telling.

Group supervision provides ways of getting in touch with what the patient brings, both said and unsaid, and what we ourselves bring to a consultation.

CASE EXAMPLE: SUE

Sue, a GP, spoke about her patient John, who had multiple medical problems and was, she felt, becoming angry and frustrated with her because she had no treatments to cure his symptoms. In the group we all noted how quickly Sue seemed to be irritated by John and his problems and when the supervisor gently asked her who John reminded her of, she thought for a few moments and then quietly said, 'He's just like my dad. I never had a good relationship with my father.' Once Sue had made this connection she was able to put aside her memories of her struggles to communicate with her father and to see John in a new and separate light.

Superimposing a difficult previous relationship onto the relationship between doctor and patient is not uncommon. In supervision we can access what may be hidden or unspoken and work towards changing entrenched patterns of behaviour both in ourselves and our patients.

A well-established group feels safe and supportive yet participants will not feel afraid to challenge, or indeed to be challenged, in a non-threatening and constructive way. The experience of seeing others make a leap of understanding and change is often the catalyst for one's own change.

For example, a confrontation between a practice manager and a salaried doctor was explored in a supervision session that I was part of. It enabled a more positive, assertive attitude from the salaried doctor. Issues of perceived powerlessness were explored and dealt with and I found this invaluable in addressing issues where I felt powerless myself. Here is an example of supervision helping with feelings of powerlessness.

CASE EXAMPLE: JASON

Jason, a salaried doctor, felt that he was always expected to work later than his contracted hours and, while he did not mind helping out at unusually busy times, it was becoming a regular occurrence for the senior partner to be away attending a meeting and for Jason to stay on to cover his patients. The senior partner told him to discuss this with the practice manager, who was always in a hurry and told him she was far too busy to see him every time she was approached. In supervision, Jason tried out phrases and body language to insist that this was a matter that needed to be sorted out and deserved time set aside to do this. It was just as high a priority as the other matters which kept the practice manager so busy. Members of the group observed Jason rehearsing with another group member playing the role of the practice manager, and with the supervisor occasionally encouraging Jason to try more powerful but positive phrases such as, 'We need to . . .', 'This situation makes me feel . . .', 'I feel that I cannot continue to work this way'. He subsequently returned to work and successfully negotiated protected time to discuss the situation productively with the senior partner and practice manager.

In supervision we are also able to recognize and understand how our patients can leave us with feelings of anger or of being taken advantage of when we have too many problems to deal with. Could this be the anger that patients are carrying with them but cannot express or even access? Is the sense of being taken advantage of exactly what patients are feeling? This process, when the supervisee carries the feelings of the patient into supervision, is a well-recognized occurrence in counselling situations, and is explored more in other chapters, particularly Chapter 2. For GPs it not only helps us to take things less personally, but gives us an opportunity to explore how patients feel and how our own inner worlds are influenced by them.

In one supervision group we acknowledged how much of our own baggage we bring to the consultation. This included a familiar sense of guilt and need to do our best for everyone, often at a personal cost to us, the doctor. Is this the sense of never being good enough that so many of us feel? Our own histories, if not acknowledged, colour a consultation. I now see how doctors can 'leak' their own issues and those from other patients into a consultation.

One useful technique that I have learnt from supervision, that helps me get in touch with my feelings and those feelings that the patients bring up for me, is to explore what I would most like to say to the patient. In the safe environment of supervision this may be spoken aloud and at times I have been surprised by what has surfaced, such as, 'I am angry with you for always taking so much time in a consultation.' Allowing me to acknowledge and notice this feeling has enabled me to work with why it is happening and both to look at strategies to manage it and let go of my frustration to enjoy more my contact with patients. Once feelings like these have been revealed and witnessed by being spoken about in supervision, the consultation with the patient frequently opens up. And even in the most challenging of cases I am able to move beyond these feelings to see and hear the patient more authentically.

Trusting my feelings was difficult at first, as I did not know how reliable they were until I had worked with them and through them for a while. I have found supervision an invaluable tool in developing my 'emotional intelligence' and have come to a point where my feelings are a reliable guide to me. I have found supervision has helped me to be fully present emotionally as well as intellectually in the consultation; it's as if my feelings provide my own internal supervisor or compass to navigate through difficult situations. I have seen others, as well as myself, become aware of their own issues, feelings and sensitivity through supervision, and use these both to manage their vulnerabilities and to perceive others (patients and colleagues) with more insight.

As the supervision groups in which I have taken part evolve, we individually and collectively start to see our own problems revealed through the person who has brought an issue. This idea of each member of a group holding or reflecting something for the group is a well-known group dynamic. The group helps to authenticate our feelings and to allow us to become more whole as a person in our relationships, not just at work but with ourselves and our families, which in turn enables others to see us fully and us to see patients more holistically.

When I talk to some doctors about supervision, they react as if the very word 'supervision' implies the supervisor being superior to the supervisee, or in some managerial position. Although this may be the case in some situations, such as in direct supervision of a junior, in the type of 'relationship' or clinical supervision that I am discussing (and that this book is about) this is rarely so. The supervisor and supervisee both learn and contribute and the relationship between them becomes a mirror of the relationship between supervisee and patient (or supervisee and colleague if that is the issue they are bringing). This mirroring if not attended to can limit the depth at which supervision takes place but when it is included in the supervision remit it provides a rich resource to both the supervisee and supervisor (see Chapter 2).

Some groups, especially those with an emphasis on support, can function perfectly well without an overall supervisor (peer groups), although most doctors will have experience of these becoming competitive or colluding. For those new to supervision, however, I would recommend trying to be part of a group with an experienced supervisor so that problems that may arise, such as difficulties in recognizing hidden emotions, are dealt with by someone with experience, who can facilitate a vital process for self-understanding (Laskowski and Pellicore 2002).

At present there seems to be considerable resistance to making time for supervision within our already over-committed days (see Chapter 12). This is entirely understandable if we only focus on the endless demands on our time or the ever full waiting room. But if we do want to examine afresh why we are challenged by something or why a feeling or situation repeats, then supervision can and does provide a breathing space to understand this. I believe that supervision has the potential to help many doctors with some of the common issues that are currently problematic to many of us in the medical profession. I see no reason why supervision cannot help others, as it has helped me.

Themes that have come up in supervision groups

Contracting

In a similar way to Balint groups, as described in Paul Sackin and John Salinsky's Chapter 3, agreement to some basic ground rules that apply to how the group runs helps to create a contained and safe space in which to supervise. These can be established at the outset but may then be revisited as supervision deepens. They may cover things like respect for all group members, confidentiality of discussions and persons discussed, time boundaries and the level of challenge and attendance.

Through my work as a supervisee, and reflecting on the supervisory agreement or 'contract', I've seen even more clearly the importance of clear, explicit working agreements and boundaries (also referred to as contracting or ground rules) to our work with patients. Failure to agree or clarify these is in my experience often at the root of difficulties for doctors and dissatisfaction of patients. In supervision I have seen a number of problems of communication between doctors and patients stem from failing to agree clearly enough the ground rules for the professional relationship between doctor and patient. The medical defence societies (Cole 2005) state that the highest number of complaints from patients are due to failure of communication and often what is not spoken aloud is as important to explore and acknowledge as what is spoken aloud. Sometimes it is easy for doctors to seem to take for granted what the 'rules of engagement' are but if these are not the ground rules the patient is working to then tensions may result. For example, a doctor who frequently runs late with a particular patient may not have been clear about the time available for the consultation. When patients' needs are not met they may develop other strategies to get what they want, e.g. if they feel they need more time or attention they may resort to complaining, petulance, demanding or even bullying tactics. When we get into difficulty in a consultation I have found it often helps to stop, go over and summarize the agreement I think we are working to and if necessary to renegotiate with the patient what I can offer and what they expect.

There may be issues surrounding confidentiality that need to be clearly stated at the outset. Patients may be afraid or misinformed about what we may or may not divulge. There may be issues with boundaries and recognizing when we or patients overstep them. I have found supervision has allowed me to practise the art of being firm with clarity and charm. For example, 'I hope you understand why we need to finish here for today', or 'This deserves a further session or longer appointment.' When I make this explicit I find working with lists that patients bring and the constraints of an appointment system much less frustrating. I have found supervision very useful in being able to rehearse how to respond in such situations, to create appropriate expectations and to give and receive feedback.

Handling uncertainty

Uncertainty is an integral part of our work. In the early stages of a doctor's career we learn certain ways to handle it, including various coping mechanisms and techniques such as safety netting. However, it often generates strong feelings and can become a cause of stress on a daily basis. It lies behind a number of issues colleagues and I have looked at in supervision. Many of us handle this informally on a day-to-day basis by 'chats' to a colleague, but it often goes unrecognized and a supervision group is a good space to identify and address recurring themes around uncertainty. Pointers I have found helpful in identifying an issue that would benefit from supervision include persistent worrying about a patient when I am at home or when I keep bringing patients back for review more frequently than colleagues, indeed whenever time and other boundaries are repeatedly broken or a patient or issue sets up strong persistent feelings.

Bereavement and endings

These can be difficult because of the depth of feelings that can be aroused in both parties. For example, a bereaved patient may trigger a doctor's own bereavement issues or a patient who has been made redundant may trigger feelings in the doctor about impending retirement or change of job.

CASE EXAMPLE: BOB

In a supervision group, Bob shared his indecision over whether it was time to retire. It emerged that he had recently been involved in a complaint and he no longer enjoyed his out-of-hours work. He was able to reflect on the emotions this had raised including fears that he was too old to think clearly and quickly enough in his job and the risks that this caused. Within a guided and supported discussion he was able to move through these emotions and the perceived feeling of loss, and acknowledge his lack of enjoyment while embracing the opportunity this reflection provided to consider retirement and the opportunities that this would provide.

This provided a chance for me to reflect on my own life choices and influences, including seeing how my desire to help patients often means that I find it difficult to entertain failure. I realized one way of looking at this is that if something hurts but does not kill me, then I emerge stronger. Supervision helps me to feel that I am not making hard decisions alone. It helps me feel I belong to the profession.

The decision to change direction of career, stop doing emergency work or consider retirement can all be discussed and explored within the supportive and confidential confines of the group – what we might call career supervision.

Abuse and support

Doctors can sometimes behave in a paternal way, which patients can experience as controlling, and patients may respond by abdicating their responsibility or challenging the doctor. If the feelings persist and deepen they might lead the doctor or patient to feel taken advantage of, sometimes obviously but at other times in subtle or hidden ways. This may manifest itself in a number of ways that can present in supervision. Sometimes quite deep issues can surface when starting from a seemingly minor issue such as looking at one's attitude to patients who miss appointments, or doctors who run late or over time.

CASE EXAMPLE

I took to supervision the case of a patient I felt had taken advantage of me. She was frequently late, often bringing multiple problems to the consultation that she knew we would struggle to deal with in the time, and made me feel manipulated and angry. She revealed in one particularly late running consultation how she had been abused by her brother both emotionally and sexually as a child, with the apparent collusion of her parents. I was initially shocked by this and struggled with guilt feelings for not being more supportive. In a supervision group I was helped to reflect honestly on my feelings and behaviour and how the feelings of guilt and inadequacy in me could help me perceive aspects of the patient's feelings. Once I was able to recognize the validity of my feelings I was able to re-engage with this patient and help her to seek further help and support.

Powerlessness

Powerlessness is an issue that I have seen come up for doctors in a number of supervision groups. In one group Peter shared a situation where he worked regularly in one practice as a salaried doctor and had been promised a regular room to work from where he could keep his equipment and books. The room had not materialized over more than six months and although he could understand the issues for the practice of time and space, he felt undervalued. When he tried to raise this it was clear that this issue was way down the list of priorities for others in the practice. The fact that his possessions lay boxed up in a cupboard contributed to him feeling like a spare part with no importance in the structure of the practice. Within the supervision group we all recognized these feelings of powerlessness in certain situations. As a group we discussed our feelings and were able to air emotions that were familiar to us all. It provided a space to reflect on the inner dialogue we have in these challenging situations and to try out different ways to express ourselves that may be less confrontational or more assertive and improve clarity of communication, changing the way we relate to others when we find ourselves in a difficult situation again.

I have come to understand that a patient who makes me feel a certain way is often projecting his or her own feelings onto me. Through supervision, including role-playing the patient, it has allowed me to explore how to manage these feelings. It may help to 'up the ante' and play up the problem to get to the root cause. In one session we explored a doctor's feelings, including fear of not being good enough. This, we were able to see, mirrored the patient's feelings, including fear that they were not good enough, and allowed us to explore ways of engaging with the patient about these feelings and how to move on.

Never good enough

This is a very common feeling among the helping and healing professions and may be what draws us to these career choices in the first place. It is often poorly understood or not recognized. The wounded healer, Chiron, in Greek mythology, is a common archetype (Cotterell 2001). Carl Jung was described as 'the wounded healer of the soul' (Dunne 2000). Jung saw Chiron as representing the healer who bears a wound that will never truly heal but who, through experience of this wound and associated pain, can become or seek to become a compassionate healer of others' wounds. We may have entered a profession to seek a way to heal ourselves. Although this is a common theme and many of us find meaning and purpose through our employment, it can be dangerous both to ourselves and our patients if not acknowledged. Many of us have encountered arrogant doctors both in real life and in popular fiction and recognize that many have personal struggles which influence the way they see and treat others. The doctor can unconsciously project such feelings onto the patient and this, if unrecognized and not dealt with by the doctor, can seriously harm the therapeutic relationship and become repeated over and over again. We may also notice that we draw a certain type of patient towards us. If we don't develop a way of coping and working with these issues, they are likely to reoccur, challenging our professionalism and even increasing our susceptibility to illness.

Acknowledging the feelings and experiences I have had through supervision has changed me and helped me in accepting who I am as the first step in this process of taking responsibility for how I work.

Themes around guilt and how good we are have recurred again and again in the supervision groups of which I have been a part. It has allowed me to revisit ideals that I have held and learn from situations when things have not gone as expected. I realize the expectations that I can cure every patient and never make mistakes are neither realistic nor healthy, and being motivated by this invites feelings of failure. Revealing and coming to understand the source of these feelings of failure (rooted in trying to fulfil unrealistic expectations) has helped free me from those expectations.

'Impostor syndrome' is not an officially recognized psychological disorder but has been much discussed in the popular press and by psychologists and counsellors. It describes those who feel that they are not worthy of their achievements and may be found out and their incompetence exposed at any stage. This may help to explain the anxieties expressed in supervision sessions and also the unease often revealed over appraisal and revalidation. A survey in a GP newspaper stated that a fifth of GPs were considering retiring rather than undergo revalidation and I wonder how many of these had a fear of being found lacking in some way (Elledge 2009). One of the ways to deal with impostor syndrome is to learn to recognize our true achievements and the effort and hard work that it has taken to reach them, and to counter the automatic negative thoughts of not being good enough. The understanding and support of a group who have already worked together for some time in a non-judgemental way, many of whom have similar feelings, enables frank discussion and a deeper understanding of how these feelings influence our choices and reactions. A supervisor should be able to distinguish between when these negative thoughts are due to the clinician's lack of confidence or competence, and when they reflect individual or collective esteem issues. Once this is clarified, an individual and group can address the feelings and an appropriate response. Working through my own feelings related to professional esteem has made me aware that I am not alone and has opened my eyes to the many doctors susceptible to feelings of inadequacy and possibly the 'impostor syndrome'.

Why supervision might be difficult (see Chapter 12)

I think many doctors feel the need to work long hours and to prove themselves. We may shy away from admitting our own fears and facing up to our issues of not being good enough. If we do not value ourselves we should not be surprised if others (colleagues and patients) do not value us. Supervision is often a challenging exercise but gives me the ability to make more conscious choices and therefore gain more control over these difficult areas. Some doctors are likely to be resistant to going against the tide and standing out or appearing different in any way. In a medical world driven by protocols and evidence-based decisions, if supervision is not seen as a routine part of one's self-development and maintaining a healthy outlook, we might not want to be seen as different from normal or too 'touchy-feely'. Valuing oneself and one's inner balance and health is not high on the priorities of many of us and, as already mentioned, the very word supervision may imply to our colleagues that we need to be watched over and further enhance the feeling of not being good enough.

What I gain from supervision

At a very basic level, attending a supervision group can be used as evidence for continuing professional development and revalidation (see Chapter 9). Attendance shows that case analysis and critical event reflection is taking place. It may also be a place to reflect on one's own health and well-being, as well as looking at our professional relationships with colleagues, and helps to prevent us becoming professionally isolated.

At a deeper level, supervision provides a supportive location for addressing the difficult areas of medical life and the many influences upon it. By giving time for reflection I gain new insight into my behaviour and reactions to challenging issues and patients. A skilled supervisor enhances this effect and draws out the hidden and less obvious factors influencing patterns of behaviour. The best supervisors need to be unafraid of challenging and addressing difficult or resisted feelings and able to recognize when the group is wandering off the point or when things become stuck. They also need to be able to hold the issues that arise and will usually be in supervision themselves.

CASE EXAMPLE

One of the most enlightening supervision sessions I have been involved in concerned a patient I had been seeing for six years and I was beginning to feel rather useless as we did not seem to be making progress. (Was this possibly mirroring the patient's feelings?) I was not sure how to move things on, so I reviewed the case notes (often a good way in itself of highlighting things you may be missing), and took the case along to supervision.

We had been stuck in the same routine every consultation. I asked how he had been doing and he gave me a long list of symptoms, unchanging, just expressed in a different way, that he hoped I would interpret for him.

A group of six of us, who had been working together in supervision alternate months over a year and had achieved an atmosphere of trust and mutual respect, discussed the case. We all felt comfortable to discuss our discomfort. Various questions came up about this patient's family relationships and particularly his relationship with his father. I had the chance to role-play a consultation twice, first playing myself, the doctor, then playing the patient. Suddenly after five minutes 'the penny dropped'. It really was as if the scales had fallen from my eyes and I could see this man in an entirely different way. Everyone had abandoned this man at varying stages in his life, beginning with his father. He had become dependent on me and fearful I would discharge (reject) him. If I told him that there was nothing more that I could do for him, this would be one more rejection, one more confirmation of his uselessness.

We rehearsed, within our supervision group, having the conversation which would move things on. I tried out the best way to raise the problem, confront the issues and reassure him that I was not going to reject him but we did need to start to discuss the real issues. This would be a real challenge for him but needed to be dealt with in order to contract to move to another level.

Once I felt comfortable with how I could raise this and how we could address progress through trying many possible scenarios, I was able to go back to my patient and successfully contract through clarification and discussion of his fears of rejection to work in more depth, having first reassured him that this would not cause further rejection. This was a real result for doctor and patient and immensely satisfying all around. The consultation had moved from being with a patient I dreaded seeing to one with whom I had a far greater rapport and understanding.

Summary

Supervision has provided me with an important insight into my struggles to enter the world of my patients and understand and work with their issues while protecting myself from over-identifying with their problems. It has helped me to recognize some of the baggage both patient and doctor are carrying. It has enabled me to face my fears about being good enough and work through my own professional issues with patients and colleagues in a safe and supportive environment. I have become a more effective communicator with patients and feel more present and at ease in what were previously difficult consultations.

My experience of supervision has highlighted areas of my work that require deeper study and reflection, allowing me to reflect on and understand my attitudes and deepen my awareness of myself and work. My way of working and, I believe, my effectiveness has been transformed by supervision. My wish in writing this chapter is that others in the medical profession may also experience this support and transformation. Supervision has helped put the enjoyment back into my work.

References

Cole, A. (2005) Complaints handling must improve in UK trusts, *BMJ*, 311: 11.
Cotterell, A. (2001) *The Encyclopaedia of Mythology*. Leicester: Anness Publishing.
Dunne, C. (2000) *The Wounded Healer of the Soul*. Sandpoint, ID: Morning Light Press.
Elledge, J. (2009) http://www.gponlinecom/News/article/908454/Exclusive-Revalidation-may-spark-GP-exodus/.
General Medical Council (2010) *Good Medical Practice*. Available at: http://www.gmc-uk.org/guidance/good_medical_practice.asp [accessed 24 May 2012].
Laskowski, C. and Pellicore, K. (2002) The wounded healer archetype: applications to palliative care practice, *American Journal of Hospice and Palliative Care*, 19(6): 403–7.

12 Listening to resistance

Robin Shohet

Editors' introduction

Resistance does not just manifest in supervision, but in encounters with patients and colleagues. The author looks at how to reframe resistance so it does not become a battle of wills, but instead seeing it as feedback on something that has not yet been understood. This requires a certain humility in each of us, to recognize that there is a different but equally valid perspective to our own and others' experiences. Realizing this increases the likelihood of co-operation not just in supervision but in any human relationship. In the context of this book this chapter explores how resistance can both serve the doctor and blind him or her to the possibility of different or new experiences. There are times when resistance needs to be honoured and others when it needs to be challenged. In understanding more about what contributes to resistance, the decision whether to honour or challenge is made easier.

Overview

Over the years of supervising, being supervised and training supervisors I have at different times and in different guises encountered resistance; resistance *to* supervision and resistance *in* supervision. In this chapter my aim is to help understand the function of resistance and, while respecting its possible value, when appropriate find skilful ways of moving beyond it. Although I am writing about resistance in the area of supervision, doctors often encounter resistance in their work with patients and many of the ideas discussed will be relevant for both situations.

Introduction

> There is something in human nature that resists being coerced and told what to do. Ironically, it is acknowledging the other's right and freedom not to change that sometimes make change possible.
>
> (Rollnick *et al.* 2008)

In this chapter, I would like to look at resistance from three different perspectives. First, I would like to look at resistance *to* supervision. If you have got this far into the book, this is unlikely to apply to you, but you may have to deal with this in those you supervise. Their resistance may not be personal but part of a wider resistance to forms of reflective practice both in the medical profession and beyond.

Most of us can resist being vulnerable, and there are times when we feel vulnerable in supervision. So from that perspective, resistance to supervision makes perfect sense.

The second perspective is looking at resistance *in* supervision, what it could mean and ways of reframing it to enable both parties to learn from it and move beyond it. I pay particular attention to whether the resistance in supervision could be mirroring the resistance that comes from the patient. Finally, once we have understood the function of resistance a little more, we can move on to practical ways of moving beyond it for the benefit of all concerned – supervisors, supervisees and patients and perhaps even the profession as a whole.

On a personal level, having supervised and been in supervision for as long as I have and felt the benefits, I was puzzled as to why it was not widespread in the medical profession. However, the more I immersed myself in relation to the medical profession and supervision, the more I began to see how little I knew. In a dialogue with a colleague she pointed out how the medical profession has managed over generations without embracing the type of supervision we are talking about in this book. Doctors have been at the coal-face of life and death issues, they have had to compete to enter medical school, to perform at an extremely high level both academically and practically, they have to communicate with people from every stratum of society and take huge responsibility on a daily basis. Why would someone with that level of experience or skill want to discuss their difficulties with a member of another profession? At this level supervision makes no sense and one would be right to resist it. But throughout the book, we have been looking at the benefits of a different approach to this one, and how there is value to all of us in sharing honestly and openly in order to solve problems. As well as anecdotal evidence, there is also empirical evidence that this can help us to perform better in our work – whoever we are (see Chapter 10 for a survey of the literature).

Core beliefs

As I started to become interested in resistance, my own and other people's, I began to see that behind the resistance were certain belief systems, often not fully conscious. I have called these core beliefs, and my experience is that these have a very strong influence on our behaviour and choices. Often resistance to supervision and in supervision is based on core beliefs. These are beliefs that are considered so self-evident that we encounter huge resistance when they are challenged. The person defending them usually does not realize they are assumptions. These beliefs determine what we see and how we process information, and can greatly contribute to the blind spots we all have. So we might have a core belief that it is rude to say what you think, which could hinder the honest exchange of views in the supervisory relationship. Or we encounter a core belief that our role in life is to take care of others. When it is suggested that doctors take care of themselves, this is seen as self-indulgent. I have come to believe that resistance often points to a core belief and this could be a very fruitful area to explore together for both supervisor and supervisee.

Every profession has its own core beliefs and it might take someone from a different profession to question some of these values. This is why we encourage a mix of professionals on our training courses, and even go as far as to suggest that supervision from different professionals can be an advantage even though they do not know the profession from the inside. After an initial discomfort (we prefer to be with people whom we consider like-minded), trainees realize how much they have to learn from each other's worlds, and how things taken for granted by one profession are not by the other. So, for example, some practitioners had very strict time boundaries, whereas others were far more flexible and each could see the advantages in the other ways of working.

Some of the core beliefs I have found to be operating in the helping professions are:

- It is my responsibility to cure the patient/client.
- I am the strong/responsible one.
- I need to know/have the answers.
- Others must come first.
- I must never make a mistake.

Sometimes questioning the validity of these core beliefs can invoke resistance, even antagonism. But if there is a willingness to explore these beliefs, we can see some of the drawbacks of holding on to them as described below.

- **It is my responsibility to cure the patient**. This denies the responsibility and resources of the patient.
- **I am the strong/responsible one**. This again denies the resources of the patient, and could stop appropriate asking for help.
- **I need to know/have the answers**. This is just not possible sometimes and is likely to contribute to stress.
- **Others must come first**. Doctors who do not take care of themselves will not be there to take care of others eventually. This is another of the core beliefs that contribute to burnout.
- **I must never make a mistake**. This is also not possible, but makes great demands on the doctor and could lead to hiding errors or unnecessary shame. This is a huge topic and is discussed in a recent book, *Being Wrong* (Schulz 2011). In relation to the medical profession, she quotes a policy of immediate acknowledging of mistakes by a hospital. The result was fewer mistakes and,

> perhaps unexpectedly, suing rates went down as patients most wanted ac-
> knowledgement more than compensation. The hospital CEO who introduced
> this policy said, 'If you don't acknowledge that mistakes occurred, you'll never
> eliminate the likelihood they will occur again' (2011: 300).

Another core belief, and one which I think applies to many of the helping professions, centres around receiving. Helman (2006) quotes cancer specialist Rachel Naomi Remen:

> One of the reason many physicians feel drained by their work is that they do
> not know how to make an opening to receive anything from their patients.
> The way we were trained, receiving is considered unprofessional. The way
> most of us were raised, receiving is considered a weakness.

Core beliefs are reinforced by the environment we find ourselves in (Realm 5 in Chapter 2), and in the case of the medical profession there can be very high expectations of a cure from the anxious patient. If doctors start to believe in their omnipotence, this may hide a fear of powerlessness which may find no place for expression, and create internal tension. Supervision can help uncover such polarities as the impotent/omnipotent ones and the price we pay for swinging between them.

Part of the reason medicine has such a strong culture is that it is dealing with some of the deepest aspects of society – the relationship to our bodies and life and death. As such the doctor can lurch between impotence (in the face of death) and omnipotence (I can cure or at least postpone death). To deal with the impotence there could be a wish for more and more certainty as a way of compensating. Tolerating uncertainty and a willingness to accept not knowing can be explored in supervision, and perhaps after initial discomfort can be a great relief.

Of course there are many other reasons for resistance – time, money, finding a suitable person are just some. However, what I have tried to do is explore some of the reasons that might relate to core beliefs in the belief that these often lie behind the more obviously rational reasons. I would now like to move on to looking at other factors that might be at play in resistance.

Contracting

The first place where we, as supervisors, might be able to work with any resistance is in the initial meeting. A clear and explicit contract can be of great value – the supervisor explaining how he or she works and what might be expected from the supervisee, who can reciprocate with his or her expectations. The supervisor might start with something like this.

> In our work together my wish is that we work collaboratively to explore issues
> that might get in the way of your fulfilling your potential and delivering the
> best service you can. This means that we can cover such topics as patients
> you might find difficult, relationships with colleagues and your practice, and

work–life balance. There are times when we might experience discomfort. This is almost invariably part of any learning process. There is a period of unlearning as we go from unconscious incompetence to conscious incompetence (where we feel most lost) to conscious competence and finally unconscious competence. I hope we will be able to talk about difficulties as they arise. What can happen is that previous experiences of feeling put on the spot can be evoked, and I hope we will be able to explore these if they come up.

Consent

Consent is crucial to the supervisory relationship. Sometimes it appears that all is going well on the surface, but underneath the supervisee has not really given consent. The supervisee might say the right things, but has not fully accepted being in supervision. This is more likely to happen if the supervisee has not chosen to be in supervision or there is an assessment or managerial function involved. In many ways this subtle resistance is harder to work with than the more obvious attacking sort. The latter is sometimes a defence against real openness and, once the storm has been weathered, I have often found that the resistant supervisee is willing to learn the most, as the example of Mark later in the chapter shows.

I have become very interested in the topics of resistance and consent and have started to run workshops with another colleague called 'Who do you bring to supervision?' This is a deliberate play on words. It is not only which patients, but how much of yourself do you feel able to bring? We explore the whole idea of a professional persona – when it is useful and when it is used to hide unnecessarily, and therefore not useful. Professional distance is usually very necessary to stop over-involvement, but can be used automatically to justify a stance that is non-relational and a chronic form of protection. Learning to monitor how we use professional distance is a very important skill that can be enhanced by supervision. The supervisor can act as a role model in showing authenticity and vulnerability as a way of countering professional distance that is used as a defence.

Control

Sometimes there might be a conscious wish to be collaborative, but the supervisor may still have an unconscious need to be in control. A possible pointer to this is resistance in the supervisee. It is easy for the supervisor to label a supervisee as resistant or difficult, but if we take the approach that resistance could be meaningful and valuable, the supervisee's resistance could be unconscious supervision about the supervisor's need to be in control. Of course it could be many other things, but we might take an approach like this: 'I am noticing that you did not want to explore such and such. I wonder if you feel I am pushing you too hard or have I not understood something about you or this case, and your reluctance is a way of telling me this? What could I have missed?' This honours apparent resistance and models non-defensiveness and a willingness to hear possible negative feedback and take responsibility for it (see Casement 1991).

Picking up cues around resistance is a very useful skill, greatly helped if the supervisor does not feel threatened. I remember a very striking instance of giving a piece of advice about how to find out about some research. At the time this was gratefully received. At the following session, the supervisee was quite subdued even though he had acted on the advice with good results. I commented on the supervisee's energy being low, and said that sometimes this means that something has happened in the previous session that contributes to this. Had I missed something perhaps, or made a mistake? The supervisee paused for a moment and then said yes. Even though the advice was useful, it had stopped him discovering how to do the research himself.

An appreciative approach

I have found it useful at the initial session with new supervisees to ask them about a good learning experience. I ask them to describe it in detail – why they thought it was good, and how we can bring some of that into our work together. This tells supervisees that our focus is going to be on strengths and successes as much as problems and tells us about their learning style. It has the effect of lowering any resistance as the feelings from the positive experience carry over into the present situation. This is part of an approach called Appreciative Inquiry (Watkins and Mohr 2011) and I will include a practical list of techniques in the summary. Many doctors might be unused to this approach, as their training involves learning to be aware of what could go wrong. While focusing on what could go wrong is of great value in terms of treatment of illness, I think it is not a good model for human relationships, where recognizing and building on strengths are of great value. Very often the key to the positive learning experience has been an important relationship, perhaps a teacher who took an interest when others didn't, and it is good to hear about this experience and learn lessons for the current relationship.

Most difficult

In training supervisors with my colleagues, we also have an opposite approach to Appreciative Inquiry and ask trainees to write down what they would find most difficult to bring to supervision and why. In this exercise, the trainee supervisor, Tom, realized he was not bringing how anxious he felt about his forthcoming appraisal. His reason was that he did not want his new supervisor to think badly of him. Once he had allowed that reason into consciousness, he realized it was not valid, and was able to take the issue to supervision with considerable benefit, as it opened up the area of fear of judgement.

Revisiting core beliefs

We have looked at core beliefs as contributing to resistance to supervision, and here is an example of core beliefs operating in both supervisor and supervisee which were temporarily affecting their ability to work together.

CASE EXAMPLE: ANN

Ann is normally quite forthcoming in supervision. She has no problems being vulnerable, owning to uncertainty, and is very open to feedback. However, in this session, when she brings her patient Mr X, she blocks suggestions the supervisor makes. The supervisor, uncharacteristically, starts to feel irritated. He has a core belief about not sharing so-called negative feelings as they could be damaging, but because of his respect for the supervisee and her usual openness, he overrides his resistance to challenge hers. He knows what is happening must mean something so says, 'I notice that uncharacteristically you are blocking me today and even more importantly I notice I am feeling irritated. I wonder if you can make sense of what is happening?' The supervisee has a lightbulb moment and replies, 'Oh my goodness. I am behaving just like my patient who says he wants help, but resists all my suggestions and even if he says yes at the time, he does not act. I am very irritated by him.' This leads to a very useful exploration of why the patient might be like that, given his family circumstances, and a compassion for him replaces her previous irritation.

The supervisor realized there was also a present time issue to explore. The supervisee had a core belief that she must like all her patients, and so it was hard for her to admit that she did not like this patient (although after the supervision this changed). The supervisor was able to overcome his resistance to sharing negative feelings and act as a role model. The supervisee was also able to recognize that having negative feelings was not something to be avoided, but a sign that could alert her to deepen her exploration of her relationship with her patients.

Understanding resistance as a form of mirroring

In this example, Ann realized that she was behaving in supervision how her patient was behaving with her. In other words, while bringing a resistant patient, supervisees become themselves resistant in supervision. This is known as mirroring or parallel process, and I have seen countless times supervisees take on their clients' behaviour when they present in supervision. Knowing about this is a very useful theoretical tool for the supervisor and can help dissolve a lot of what appears or gets acted out as resistance.

Resistance arising from differences in culture

Here is an example from general practice.

CASE EXAMPLE: AZIZ

Aziz was from a middle eastern culture and always asked about a patient's family, took great interest in them, and remembered their details. He was very popular with patients, but was seen as very inefficient by other doctors because he often overran. Core beliefs in the value of family context, and taking time for this, were in conflict with the values of efficiency. These needed to be teased out in supervision so he could see more clearly his fellow practitioners' point of view and make more informed choices. This had benefits for all parties.

Reframing as a way of working with resistance

What can sometimes happen, especially if supervisees feel that they did not have a choice about their supervisor or having supervision, is that they might agree intellectually, but not change their behaviour. In this case the supervisor will need to listen carefully to the resistance. The supervisor could ask himself and then his supervisee what he (the supervisor) has not yet understood, or check out if the supervisee feels she is being required to behave or think differently – in other words, reframe the resistance of the supervisee in terms of what the supervisor might or might not be doing. To show that this applies beyond supervision, those of us who have children can see this when we get apparent agreement from them to, say, tidy their rooms. When this is not done, rather than be angry we can realize that the agreement was actually still our trying to control. A useful skill of the supervisor is to be able to reframe a situation, as the following example will illustrate, where the supervisor reframed a complaint into a commitment. The supervisor is using commitment in a particular way to illustrate a commitment to a belief that a feeling, in this case anger, might have been masking.

CASE EXAMPLE: JOHN

In a supervision group, John was often late and one of the group members in particular was gearing up to a confrontation. The supervisor said that perhaps the anger was pointing to a commitment and, rather than expressing anger, what might the commitment be? The supervisee paused and then said, 'This group is such a valuable resource for me. I want us all to be able to share it together.' Once this had been elicited the supervisee was able to share this with the latecomer in a much softer way which was not resisted, whereas previous challenges had been met with resistance in the form of excuses.

An amusing example of reframing with patients is given by Helman (2006). The author describes working in a stockbroker belt with high powered patients who had very self-destructive habits. They were driven, obsessed with deadlines, rushing, tense. Telling them all of this and how it might damage their health simply didn't work ... but phrase it in their language and their ears would prick up:

Why don't you see your health, and your body as your capital. And see stopping smoking as an investment, a long-term investment. One that in a few years will earn you a high rate of interest. Just think of all those dividends. It's an investment that is bound to pay off. Invest in your body now and think of all those profits in years to come!

(Helman 2006: 77)

In the following example the reframing was done by recognizing a competing commitment which was inhibiting the supervisee from acting.

CASE EXAMPLE: AMY

Amy, a junior doctor, felt she was being bullied by the senior partner, but resisted any suggestions as to what she might do about it. The supervisor wondered in a very non-judgemental way if she could share what might be stopping her from taking the action she wanted to take, and challenging her boss. Perhaps there was something of real value that was even more important than challenging her boss (the competing commitment). Amy was puzzled and the supervisor hinted that perhaps the fear of being emotional and therefore weak could be present. There might be a commitment to her self-respect that was greater than her need to challenge. Amy was able to resonate to this and together they explored whether being emotional was in fact weakness, however it was perceived. Finding the competing commitment, i.e. seeing there was a conflict between wanting to challenge and fearing being vulnerable, helped to dissolve the resistance. Simply giving strategies for tackling the senior partner might not have worked as well.

Finding the commitment in the complaint/resistance

Many of us when faced with a complaint are likely to become defensive. In the following example the supervisor was able to model a different way of working with a complaint by finding the commitment in the complaint.

CASE EXAMPLE: MARK

Mark makes it clear that he thinks supervision is a waste of time. He has managed very well for the last fifteen years without it. He says that the last group, especially, was a complete waste of time. People just talked and talked about themselves mainly, and even when they did talk about the patient, it was mostly speculation instead of sticking to the facts. The supervisor, at this point, could have become defensive around the complaint, but sees the commitment in the resistance. She says that she hears that he is committed to making good use of time, with which he agrees. She adds that she knows that the welfare of the patient is important to him, to which he impatiently replies, 'Of course.' So, she continues, bringing these together, a group that really focuses on the well-being of the patient in an efficient way might be useful? He agrees and adds that a training group where he could learn up-to-date methods and the latest research would be a far better use of his time. The supervisor says she can well understand this, but would he be willing to present a case to the group and see how it felt to be on the receiving end of the supervision? He doubtfully agrees and the group uses a technique of all asking one question which could take the work further, which he was not to answer then, but write down and think about. Mark is quite surprised at how useful it has been, giving perspectives he had not thought about. He says that he had been taught that when he had difficulties to get on with things and put it all to the back of his mind, and that he was too old to change now. The following week he brings the case of a woman patient who had been getting on his nerves and says with a smile, '... and don't go telling me she reminds me of my mother.' The group role-plays different ways of approaching her while the supervisee watches quite thoughtfully and says how useful it has been. Here the skill of recognizing the commitment in the complaint and the apparent competing commitments (efficiency and welfare of patients) was important in overcoming the resistance. In this way she was able to reframe how the group could work for Mark.

Resistance protecting vulnerability and the courage to go beyond

In supervision there can often be resistance to feeling vulnerable, the core belief being that it is a sign of weakness. The supervisor might feel frustrated when he or she sees signs of not coping which the supervisee adamantly denies. Understanding that there might be core beliefs operating around not appearing weak will help the supervisor come alongside the supervisee more easily.

A supervisor can often forget how vulnerable it makes people feel to go to supervision and talk about issues that are difficult – whether it be patients or colleagues or difficulties at home that are leaking into work. In my supervision work I encounter a real fear in supervisees of being shamed, to which the supervisor needs to be sensitive. This is especially true of group situations and a group supervisor needs to know a lot about group dynamics (the Balint groups are well structured to help minimize the less co-operative side of groups and bring in the co-operative – see Chapter 3). I believe it is important that supervisors themselves be willing to experience their own vulnerability and, if appropriate, share it with the supervisee.

There is a school of thought that says that people with whom we are uncomfortable can be our teachers, showing us aspects of ourselves that we might not normally encounter. If we can't accept they have something to offer us, however, we will avoid, blame and try and find others to collude with our negative opinions of those who seem to create our discomfort. Supervision can help us learn to go past our natural resistance to sticking with uncomfortable feelings which make us feel vulnerable, and I have been witness to this process of potential transformation many times (Shohet 2011, Chapter 11).

A model I have found useful in mapping out the levels of helping, which I found in a book called *The Courage to Teach* (Palmer 1998), is to distinguish the what, the how, the why and the who of a profession. Applying this to medicine, the what is the disease and diagnosis, the how is the treatment (Realm 1, Chapter 2), the why is questioning some of the norms and core beliefs around medicine (Realm 5, Chapter 2), and the who is looking at the person of the doctor and what he or she brings into the consultation (Realm 3, Chapter 2). It is the last two that are the real focus of supervision we are writing about in this book. I regularly witness in supervision the courage to examine core beliefs and blind spots, and a willingness in supervisees to look at themselves, but can also empathize with the resistance to doing this. In our training groups we do an exercise looking at how participants might sabotage their learning, for example by withdrawing or feeling critical or not good enough. It is very interesting to share these, a way of anticipating the resistance, as we all have at least some of these behaviours or scripts. This exercise can be done in the supervisory relationship, too, looking at and naming the potential pitfalls. Once the possibility of resistance occurring has been named, it seems to make it less likely to happen, or for it to happen without awareness.

To challenge or not

At this stage we need to ask ourselves when is it useful to go along with resistance until the relationship is on a more secure footing, and can be challenged later; when is it a sign that something is wrong and the resistance is a healthy refusal to go along with that, the psychic equivalent of the immune system; and when does it need to be pushed through – and how do we recognize the difference? I have no ready answers to such questions, but would remind you of the technique mentioned earlier of supervisors asking if there is something they have missed or not understood. As well as showing a non-defensive stance, it gives an opportunity for supervisees to share what they might not have consciously realized was bothering them.

Hawkins and Shohet (2006: 212–13), in their chapter on developing supervision policy and practice in organizations, look at resistance to change in organizations. They quote many reasons that apply personally as well as organizationally such as fear of the unknown, lack of information, no perceived benefits, threat to status, reluctance to experiment. They quote the work of Kurt Lewin (1952), who adapted from physics into the field of human relations the law that says: 'Every force creates its equal and opposite force.' Hawkins and Shohet write, 'If the resistance can be honoured and redirected, the change will happen without having to use greater effort' (2006: 213).

In the following example the group tried to push through the resistance, which only increased it, and the supervisor was able to recognize this and redirect it.

CASE EXAMPLE: BETH

In a group supervision, the members were challenging a group member, Beth, quite forcibly about an issue about breaking confidentiality. The supervisor agreed with their challenge, but not the way they were doing it, as the supervisee was getting more and more uncomfortable. He said, 'I notice that the group is being very challenging to you, Beth. When this happens it sometimes means that the group is not taking responsibility for how they might have done, or could do, what you have done. You are reminding them that at some stage they might have done what you did, or fear that they might do in the future.' The group agreed and apologized to Beth, who was then able to explain her competing commitment to confidentiality but also to the welfare of the family as she saw it, and that she had in fact made a mistake.

Wilful blindness. Resisting group norms

Resistance does not only apply to supervision, as we can all find areas of our lives where we resist. In a book called *Wilful Blindness* (Hefferman 2011) the author describes how we do not want to see anything which threatens our world view, what I have called our core beliefs in this chapter. We may consciously think we can appreciate difference, but she quotes evidence to show that we choose friends, partners, neighbourhoods where our comfort around similarity is not threatened. Where this gets dangerous or dysfunctional is when we choose to ignore the evidence in order to manage a competing commitment to belong. There are classic psychological experiments, starting with the classic experiments of Asch (1951), that show people will report seeing lines longer than they are because the rest of the group appear to think the same (the other members of the group are stooges). The need to belong, not to rock the boat, is very strong, so we have to make a conscious commitment to go for truth rather than comfort. Supervision, if it is going to be valuable, will help us uncover blind spots, and this may not always feel comfortable, especially when it means not going along with the group norms. As such, it may be useful for supervisors to be in a different profession because they have an outside perspective and may not be party to the same core beliefs. There are arguments for and against a supervisor coming from the same profession, but outsiders do have something to offer as they can question the norms and core beliefs of the profession more easily.

Summary

Resistance can potentially provide both supervisor and supervisee with very useful information. It can point to unhelpful core beliefs on a personal and professional level, and these can be explored in supervision. I believe it plays an important part in the medical profession from the patient upwards, and as such is worthy of attention. There are no easy answers as to when to honour the resistance and when to challenge it, but my approach has been that listening carefully to the resistance can deepen the learning for both parties.

My wish is not just to give ways of listening and insight, but also practical tools, and I have summarized them below.

- Clear contracting to explain the purpose of supervision, the way of working and sharing expectations.
- Sharing positive experiences of supervision and learning.
- When noticing resistance, supervisors being willing to check themselves out to see if they have missed something rather than blame the supervisee.
- Eliciting and making explicit core beliefs.
- Reframing – seeing the commitment behind the complaint.
- Noticing competing commitments and making them explicit.
- Recognizing parallel process whereby supervisees begin to present in the same way as their patient has presented to them. In other words, recognizing that the resistance can go from patient, to supervisee, to supervisor.
- Naming the potential for sabotage right at the beginning.

My belief is that resistance, like the immune system, is there for a purpose and we need to understand it and work with it, especially in those instances where it can put the body on false alert. Extending the analogy, supervision can be seen as a way of enhancing the body's immune system, with similar great benefits in helping to stop, or at least reduce, the prevalence of the 'dis-ease' of stress and burnout and promoting a healthier life style.

Acknowledgements

To Christina Breene, whose chapter in *Supervision as Transformation* (Shohet 2011) gave me the idea for this chapter.

References

Asch, S. E. (1951) Effects of group pressure upon the modification and distortion of judgment, in H. Guetzkow (ed.) *Groups, Leadership and Men*. Pittsburgh, PA: Carnegie Press.
Casement, P. (1991) *On Learning from the Patient*. New York: Guilford Press.
Hawkins, P. and Shohet, R. (2006) *Supervision in the Helping Professions*. Maidenhead: Open University Press.
Hefferman, M. (2011) *Wilful Blindness*. New York: Simon and Schuster.
Helman, C. (2006) *Suburban Shaman*. London: Hammersmith Press.
Lewin, K. (1952) Defining the field at any given time, in D. Cartwright (ed.) *Field Theory in Social Science*. London: Tavistock.
Palmer, P. (1998) *The Courage to Teach*. Chichester: John Wiley.

Rollnick, S., Miller, W. and Butler, C. (2008) *Motivational Interviewing in Health Care.* New York: Guilford Press.

Schulz, K. (2011) *Being Wrong: Adventures in the Margin of Error.* London: Portobello Books.

Shohet, R. (2011) *Supervision as Transformation. A Passion for Learning.* London: Jessica Kingsley Publishers.

Watkins, J. M. and Mohr, B. J. (2001) *Appreciative Inquiry.* Chichester: John Wiley.

Index

Locators shown in *italics* refer to case examples, tables and figures.

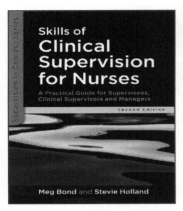

SKILLS OF CLINICAL SUPERVISION FOR NURSES
Second Edition

Meg Bond and Stevie Holland

9780335238156 (Paperback)
2011

eBook also available

This perennial bestseller provides a practical and accessible, skills-based text on how to implement and engage in clinical supervision. It provides clear frameworks to guide learning, with real-life examples from across the range of nursing specialisms.
Offering grounded perspectives on supervision for nurses, it has been thoroughly updated to reflect changes and developments in the profession.

Key features:

- Exploration of the theory and development of clinical supervision
- An analysis of the process and skills of in-depth reflection
- Guidelines on developing key skills for both supervisors and supervisees

www.openup.co.uk

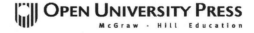

OPEN UNIVERSITY PRESS
McGraw · Hill Education

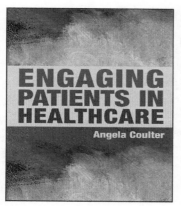

ENGAGING PATIENTS IN HEALTHCARE

Angela Coulter

9780335242719 (Paperback)
2011

eBook also available

This new text is a complete guide to patient engagement and participation in healthcare, which is a central theme of health policy in the UK and internationally. Angela Coulter explains the theories, models and policies used as well as giving extensive practical examples to illustrate the reality of patient involvement, and how it impacts on health outcomes. Based on 250 systematic reviews in the area, this is the most current and comprehensive text on the market.

Key features:

- Full of practical examples from the UK and abroad
- Provides an excellent overview of patient engagement
- Written by a leading author in the field

www.openup.co.uk

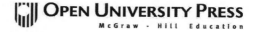

OPEN UNIVERSITY PRESS
McGraw - Hill Education

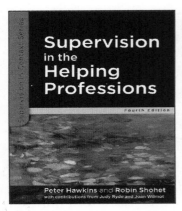

**SUPERVISION IN THE HELPING
PROFESSIONS**
Fourth Edition

Peter Hawkins and Robin Shohet

9780335243112 (Paperback)
2012

eBook also available

This bestselling book provides a comprehensive guide to supervision for
professionals across the social care and helping professions, as well as those
working in education, coaching and human resources. Thoroughly updated, the
book has a new introduction showing how the world context in which helping
professions operate has fundamentally changed in the last 25 years and the
implications of this for supervision.

Key features:

- The CLEAR model for structuring the process of a supervision session
- How to adapt supervision to learning styles
- How to use video and interpersonal process recall in training supervisors

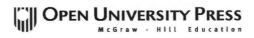

www.openup.co.uk